"In Our Professional Opinion . . ."
The Primacy of Clinical Judgment
over Moral Choice

"In Our Professional
The Primacy of

Opinion . . ."
Clinical Judgment over Moral Choice

Wendy Carlton

University of Notre Dame Press

Notre Dame   London

Library of Congress Cataloging in Publication Data

Carlton, Wendy, 1949–
 "In our professional opinion . . ."

  Bibliography: p.
  Includes index.
  1. Medical education—Social aspects—United States.
2. Medical students—United States. 3. Medicine—
Decision making. 4. Medical ethics. 5. Professional
socialization. I. Title.[DNLM: 1. Ethics,
Medical. 2. Students, Medical. 3. Socialization.
W50.3 C285i]
R745.C26   301.5   78-51524
ISBN 0-268-01143-5

For
My Parents,
Robert and Lucille Carlton

Contents

Preface

This book grew out of a research seminar in field methods with Doctors Renée Fox and Jerold Starr. Motivated by Dr. Fox's longstanding interest in the professional socialization of medical students, I decided to investigate how the contemporary medical student has changed since the days of *The Student-Physician*.[1] It was Dr. Fox's opinion that "the data needed to resolve the question, 'Is there a "new" medical student?' are lacking. But those who believe and those who disbelieve are reacting to the same phenomena."[2]

Other influences include the development of a literature on death and dying, and the founding in 1969 of the Institute of Society, Ethics and the Life Sciences (The Hastings Center).[3] It may be said that the work of Elizabeth Kübler-Ross served as a catalyst for my own thinking and for that of other sociologists who became concerned with the interrelationships between the social sciences and medicine.[4] This concern has spurred discussion and debate of topics that have been subsumed under the rubric bio-ethics.[5] The renewed interest in the application of ethics to the practice of medicine was indicative of a shift of focus brought about by the increasingly technological aspects of medicine. Whether bio-ethics has an existence independent of the academic disciplines that contribute to its literature, such as philosophy, law, and sociology, is not of concern here. Rather, I want to convey the climate of interest which supported consideration of ethical questions in the clinical setting.

A university hospital located in a large midwestern city was selected as the primary research site because it was accessible through the good offices of a medical sociologist who shall remain unnamed. Little will be said of its location or physical plant, in order to increase the prospects of anonymity. Pseudonyms have been given to all participants, and some identifying clues have been deliberately changed.

Styles of sociological research are diverse; they encompass historical materials, mathematical models, communication-oriented methodologies such as the interview and the questionnaire, and techniques borrowed from anthropology that are called "field methods."[6] Research methods and research demands must be congruent. Participant observation was selected for this study because it seemed appropriate to the information goal.[7] It would allow me to get at the physicians' management of decision-making so that I could develop insight into their problem perspective without forcing them to conform to my preconceptions of how physicians behave. It would allow me to tap behavior which is not included in their oral or written accounts of how decisions are made. When asked how they make decisions, physicians tend to give very simplistic answers or to argue that it is "second nature—like walking or talking." Their written accounts of decision-making, the hospital charts, are frequently missing many details or written with a particular audience in mind, such as the hospital review committee, which evaluates length of patient stay. Also, charts are sometimes written weeks after the patient has left the floor, and the charts themselves are sometimes lost. Participant observation would allow me access to the daily behavior which contains the social clues to doctors' overall perspective—the jargon, the jokes, and the institutional pressures which became incorporated into a professional posture. Finally, it would allow me to construct a typology which could account for the absence as well as the presence of phenomena.

It was a condition of my participation on the pediatrics service that I be formally introduced to the parents of patients in order to receive their participation. On all other services it was handled informally. I was introduced by the resident or attending physicians as "a member of our team" and occasionally as "our sociologist." The medical student always introduced me to the patient he was to examine or to care for.

My presence in the clinical setting was an important research tool. Since I wanted to pick up the implicit cues and instructions which are communicated to students independent of the medical content of discussion, I needed to be there when decisions were being made. I was also concerned with how I might obtain data with the least resistance and with the fewest overt demands on students and house officers (interns and residents). Both physicians and students disapproved of questionnaires and formal interview schedules, but were genuinely interested in, sometimes almost perplexed by, my nearly constant attendance. For despite the fact that I was not always present for their sometimes eighty-hour weeks, I was there on the service for longer stretches of time than a medical student would expect of a sociologist.

There were additional advantages. Through participant observation I got to observe a great number of people in their natural setting with minimal contact with bureaucratic channels of authority. I did not have to get permission from all the consulting services, visiting attending physicians, and auxiliary personnel in order to tap their contributions and their knowledge. Similarly, I was not limited to persons who would be willing to submit to formal interviews. I could take refuge in being a member of the team. Finally, I frequently rendered myself invisible through the posture I adopted, thus acquiring information that would not otherwise have been available to me.

There were disadvantages, too. Participant observation is time-consuming and physically exhausting. The hours are long, and the number of sprints down the stairs to the labs and back up to the floor can be countless. It is not conducive to development and elaboration, since it does not allow the researcher to prod and develop a sequence of ideas as an interviewer with an organized schedule of questions can. It is much more akin to extemporaneous theater, where the actor seizes an opportunity with an eye half-cocked in the direction of the next possibility. It requires the development and breaking off of relationships, with a large emotional component of loss. In spending many, many hours with one student there is the opportunity of forming an intense relationship which is then abruptly terminated by the requirements of the calendar. On a less personal level, participant observation has the drawback of tentative reliability. It is not so easily replicable as is research based on attitudinal scales, questionnaires, or formal interviewing. In this study, a degree of internal consistency arose across services, and I checked my observations against those of students and house staff to integrate their responses into my descriptive accounts. Nevertheless, until other sociologists develop this area further, the reliability of my sociological analysis rests with me and whatever collaborative documentation I can incorporate.

The general plan of my research was to follow a medical student as he fulfilled the requirement of his clinical elective. These were four-week rotations, and each month both the service and the student changed. This occurred eight times. Each semester I submitted a list of requests for rotations to the dean of students, and he recruited willing informants who then contacted me.

Although there are several medical centers affiliated with University Medical School, students were selected from those taking electives at University Hospital and Children's Hospital. The latter was included because the decision to specialize in "medicine" versus pediatrics was considered to be an important milestone in professional socialization.

The dean was asked to limit the informants to third- and fourth-year male students. Upper-class students were chosen because they are not subject to the heavy lecture schedules of first- and second-year students. Upper-class students participate full time in clinical programs and acquire increasingly heavy responsibility for patients as they progress toward a degree. Observations of second-year students were based on a preliminary study I had performed and on their presence on services which also had upper-class externs, such as pediatrics, medicine, and psychiatry. The limitation on gender was imposed because the classic studies of medical students were concerned only with male students.[8] I did not want variations from those initial observations attributed to the use of female students as informants.

As I went into the field I worried that I would be studying the deviants of the medical school, the nonaggressive, humanistic aberrations who would not feel threatened by the presence of a sociologist. Over the course of several months I learned that this fear was unfounded. Informants were well socialized into their institutional roles. Several of them announced at the start of a rotation, "You wait and see. I'll ask some ethical questions before the rotation is over." This happened very rarely, and not without institutional stimulus, such as the presence of an attending physician who headed the Patients' Rights Committee. The informants varied in their professional goals, from wanting to be "a good country doc" to hoping to excel in cardiology, an exceptionally high-pressured clinical specialty. Their interests were in medicine and pediatrics rather than surgery, so I am ill equipped to comment on how future surgeons differ from these young men. Some were smarter and more capable than others, but by their own accounts they were neither the best nor the worst of their respective classes. Although I can claim to know fewer than a dozen students intimately, I came to know many other students, interns, and residents through them in the course of sharing meals, seeing consulting teams, and touring the halls. A conservative estimate would be that one hundred and fifty people appear in my field notes as somehow contributing to my understanding of the clinical perspective. As time went on, the students I followed became a network known to each other, so that I was increasingly spared the need to explain and justify my presence to the degree that had at first been necessary. The fact that people had seen me around aided my identification as "one of us."

The use of participant observation and auxiliary skills of interviewing, document-collecting, and extensive reading of both sociological and medical materials allowed me to let my material shape my thesis, rather than artificially impose order on acquired data. What started out as a study of the socialization of medical students to decision-making became a complex study of the limited, almost nonexistent, socialization of medical students to ethical issues in clinical practice. In the early months of fieldwork I became convinced of the need to delineate a fundamental context in which ethical situations intrude in order to talk with any sensitivity of the problems of physicians. While I might have concerned myself with three *realities*—the physician's, the layperson's, and the sociologist's—I instead found that physicians use one or more perspectives which may overlap with those of other observers in a clinical setting. Hence, I found it useful to talk about three *perspectives:* the clinical, the legal, and the moral. By sampling physicians' routines, I learned that their definition of *reality* is an organizational construct which allows them to make the clinical reality manageable and bearable. They are selecting from among three perspectives on problem-solving, rather than ascribing to a monolithic "reality."

The limitations of qualitative methods must be acknowledged, as well as the limits of my own skills. The conclusions drawn from one university teaching hospital cannot be taken as evidence of what occurs at all teaching hospitals.[9] The generalizations of this study are limited to medical services in University Hospital. Within the boundaries of its own limitations, it is submitted as an accurate depiction of the acquisition of perspective in medical training and practice. The subordinate thread is the socialization of a sociologist; the one does not exist without the other.[10]

Acknowledgments

Many people who helped in significant ways must remain nameless; without their cooperation there would be no book. The following people can be thanked publicly for their assistance during various phases of writing, rewriting, and editing: Dr. Ann Beuf, Dr. Otto Pollak, and Dr. Harold Bershady, all of the University of Pennsylvania; Dr. Stanley Hauerwas, University of Notre Dame; and Jim Langford, director of the University of Notre Dame Press. I also appreciate the help of Phyllis Padow and my husband, Mark Needleman.

Introduction

College students pursue admission to medical school like knights charging toward Camelot. They are confident that both personal satisfaction and financial reward await them. Neither Marcus Welby, M.D., nor local luminaries in the medical profession dispel the illusion of the quest. Not even the grinding endurance test known as the first two years of medical school dispels the idealism, for inside every exhausted student is a "dedicated physician" waiting to be born. It is not until their first clinical rotations that medical students are exposed to the pressures which impinge on physicians' actions. The demands of peers, hospital administrators, community politicians, and patients become apparent to students who once thought that the practice of medicine consisted exclusively of healing and curing. As students progress through assorted tests of professional identity, they find that they are not always certain what they are seeking, nor is the way clearly marked.

Juxtaposed against the idealistic young are their more chary role models, the academic clinicians. Some have long ago lost the vision of Camelot and content themselves with a limited range of medical problems and an expansive income. Many of these teachers continue to speak warmly of medicine as a profession, enumerating the satisfaction of "solving mysteries" and of seeing patients get better under their care. A select few have incorporated a holy awe of medicine into their professional selves, speaking of the "wisdom of the body" and urging their students to see themselves as the handmaidens of nature.

Among these competing visions of medicine stand diverse notions of "the good," the values physicians strive to fulfill, as well as

1

the means to their satisfaction. This generation of elder physicians, however, frequently finds that the old rules of how and when to act are not applicable or, when applied, fail to make sense. A review of earlier literature demonstrates no systematic instruction in responding to the problems that medical technology creates, such as when to disconnect respirators or how to select patients for "random clinical trials."[1] To date, the practice of medicine has required the determination of clinical status and one of two choices: the selection of appropriate therapy or the confrontation with the reality that no therapy exists. Increasingly, physicians face an ambiguous third alternative. They can treat an acute problem which appears to be life-threatening, but can do nothing to halt the patient's overall trajectory toward death. Where there is no promise of repair or recovery, there is a need to consider whether such "treatment" is appropriate to the patient's needs.

The dilemmas founded in this third alternative frequently invoke rules of action that are tied to moral notions of "right" and "wrong," but are not tied to any overarching ethical system. In other words, there is an apparent lack of moral consensus which might locate these kinds of decisions within a system of rules that both physicians and laypersons could apply. Since contemporary social life is only loosely linked to a secular ethical system, physicians as well as laypersons tend to cope with the ethical dilemmas on a case-by-case basis, using the fragmentary moral rules as a substitute for the universal rules they lack.

Quite frequently the premises and conclusions relevant to an individual case can be evaluated without seeking to generalize to other situations and without searching for precedents.[2] For example, a physician may hold that no care need be given to an elderly patient who has advanced cancer; thus he or she will not advocate extensive antibiotic therapy when that patient contracts pneumonia. The assumption here is that treatment of the pneumonia will extend suffering, and the minimization of suffering is a stronger obligation than that of extending life for a few days or weeks. Yet, even if we accept this argument and the conclusion to offer no care, we find ourselves with little basis to examine the question of caring for a defective newborn with marked mental disability but no marked physical handicaps. Though it may still be argued that an obligation exists to minimize suffering while refraining from any direct action of killing, one cannot readily generalize to the second situation. Furthermore, it would be most unusual for the physician to research clinical precedent relevant to each of these situations, though he or she may be acquainted with what colleagues have done in similar situations. For the most part, each situation is treated as a bounded proposition, requiring simply the clinical facts at hand for each of the respective patients. This lopping off of "extraneous" information is an important part of clinical decision-making, which is exaggerated in the context of examining how physicians cope with ethical dilemmas.

The need to evoke case-by-case review and the de facto isolation of the premises and conclusions from any kind of moral principles, either secular or sacred, ties the physician to a system of situational ethics that is based in professional consensus. The assumption of congruence between the values of physicians and those of laypersons is founded on the illusion of consistency between personal and professional morality—namely, that John Doe, M.D., would make identical decisions acting in his capacity as a physician as he would as a father, husband, or friend. The discontinuity between these roles and their value assumptions is a major contributor to the antagonism between physicians and laypersons.

Even when physicians act in a manner consistent with "the standards of clinical practice," they are still open to criticism as well as to the possibility of malpractice litigation. Fears of being legally culpable have created a form of practice known as "defensive medicine." Medical students are being taught that they should order tests and x-rays for "medical-legal" reasons in order to document a comprehensive investigation of the complaint for which the patient was admitted. This leads to inflated expense as well as to medical conservatism, neither of which is in the interest of the patient. Some physicians, aware of this legal trap, may contend that their decisions are founded on a broad substratum of clinical judgment and personal experience which reflects moral precepts of what is "right." This honorable position, however, affords little protection from abuse. For the questions are too new, too complex, and too weighty to simplify themselves with reference to professional ethics or civic morals.

In the light of these difficulties, many people hold that medical students should be taught ethical theory as part of the medical school curriculum and then be provided with formal opportunities to apply philosophical tools to clinical cases in order to become sensitized to the ethical issues inherent in their clinical responsibility. As the arguments unfold, I shall make a case for the futility of using the classroom to remedy these problems. My research denies me a basis for such optimism and simplicity. I shall argue that without radical changes in the structure of hospital bureaucracy and in the delegation of professional authority by physicians, medical students and house officers on university medical services will continue to limit their professional focus to clinical detail and the incumbent responsibilities of medical management. This limitation is reinforced by the absence of role models who act consistently within the norm of "ethical concern." Thus, students learn to disregard questions of values.

The obliqueness of physician attention to so-called ethical issues is not a function of stupidity or ignorance, which would require educational remediation, or simply of abuse of professional prerogatives, which would necessitate supervision by some regulatory body, such as a PSRO (Professional Standards Review Organization). It is founded on institutional constraints which reinforce certain kinds of behavior that have been elicited and rewarded throughout professional training. Furthermore, it is tied to an ideology which reinforces the status quo by discouraging the recruitment of individuals who would not readily conform to the institutionalized role dictated by the pursuit of collegial acceptance.

The student who expects to incorporate humanism into medicine, who swears to be morally upright throughout the medical novitiate, frequently finds that in order to satisfy a definition of a "good" student or physician he or she must sacrifice one or both of these aspects of performance in order to fulfill an ideal of rationality and efficiency. While humanism may translate into a concern for men and women who are sick (as opposed to a concern for the illnesses of patients),[3] it is not synonymous with attention to the moral underpinnings of medicine. Yet without the former, the latter probably will not appear. As Charles Fried points out, one cannot uphold a standard of personal care if the scope of attention is limited to a diseased organ or to the opportunity for study of clinical exotica.[4]

I have already suggested that the pursuit of a definition of "ethical concern" founded in universal moral rules is quixotic. This naive belief in a set of moral rules which could illuminate the ethical problem and resolve the ethical dilemma is tempting. While many philosophers have concerned themselves with the properties of moral ideas, it is outside the expertise and competency of this sociologist to do justice to the problem. Without my experiences in the field, I might still cling to the assumption that the identification of the implicit moral rules would clarify human behavior regardless of the professional status of the actor or the object of the action. If this were the case, then resolution of professional limitation could be served by elaborating on the rules and the means by which they are invoked. How simple it seems behind the typewriter, how difficult on the clinical service.

What interests the sociologist is why the boundaries of the moral universe vary with respect to the kinds of behavior and the status of the actors rather than to particular approaches to the rules of ethical analysis. Within sociology there is a long tradition of concern with moral life. As an extreme view one might be tempted to argue that all human behavior contains ethical propositions because it is founded on normative expectations which contain notions of what is "right" and what is "desirable." This, however, is a meaningless stance. It tells us nothing about how the rules of "rightness" and "desirability" are determined, nor does it give us any insight into those categories of action which are implicitly identified as part of "morality" and those which are assumed under a more general rubric of "human behavior." Any discussion of killing, for example, evokes discussion of its moral grounding. The mere mention of killing elicits "ethical concern." On the other hand, there are some categories of behavior, as, for example, the study of astrophysics, which are treated as if they were morally neutral, when in fact, even if only implicit in this "pure knowledge," there are applied uses that are rife with moral outcomes.[5] A third category of actions seems to be totally outside moral analysis, such as brushing one's teeth. While I suppose a case for oral hygiene could be founded on the ideal of health as a moral "good," this implicit argument would be obscure to all but a handful of professors. It would fail to explain the identity of health as a "good," or to explain why the implicit moral argument has so little salience in the decision to brush one's teeth. In this third situation, morality seems irrelevant; in the second, it awaits the misuse of knowledge; in the first, it demands recognition.

The physician and the student physician are plunged into a social setting which consists of patient, physician, and medical institution. They do not share identical value systems, nor do they have the same authority to evoke and to pursue their differences. Unless one of the parties to a clinical decision makes explicit the lack of value consensus, as when the patient asserts religious beliefs, the illusion of consensus will be assumed and maintained. In particular, the physician's judgment of what is in the best interest of the patient will be offered and accepted, unless the patient or the hospital administrator is prepared to challenge the physician.

As much as physicians hate being wrong, they seem to find even more devastating the prospect of not knowing what to do. The existence of numerous problems which paralyze their inclinations to do something, and at the same time threaten them with the possibility of being wrong, does little to enhance their security and self-confidence. Furthermore, they know that if nonphysicians could find an effective voice to assert that physicians are no better trained or educated to handle ethical dilemmas than comparably educated laypersons, then the guise of their self-assurance would be exposed. Their ambivalence and their lack of understanding would become a public matter, no longer tied to the protective insulation of their collegial networks. Such exposure might ultimately mean that laypersons would want to share in these difficult decisions; yet physicians seem determined to extend their authority over vast areas of professional practice, even when other professionals and paraprofessionals might relieve them of some of the unnecessary burden.

At first there appears to be an irresolvable conflict between those who recommend expanding the scope of authority and responsibility of physicians and those who favor restricting that scope. On the one hand, tied to the hue and cry against amoral physicians and their lack of concern for the "whole person" is a program of change which entails increasing responsibility and increasing their domain of jurisdiction. On the other hand, the opposing tactic, to curtail their responsibilities and to limit their authority, appears to move them closer to the image of mere technicians, which few people would regard as a desirable alternative.

My own thinking reflects this conflict. When I started out in the field, I thought the physician ought to be committed first and foremost to the well-being of the patient. Other interests, such as particular facets of the case which are important in clinical research, might be served in the course of treatment. In view of this concern, I believed that the physician should consider the patient as an individual rather than as a set of organ systems.[6] It is the physician's concern with the well-being of the individual that the public readily identifies as the trait of a "good doctor." So as I began my research I favored the "whole person" position, arguing that the physician is obligated to pursue the interest of the person, rather than to substitute goals of research investigation or professional advancement.[7] Indeed, the University Medical School catalogue alludes to this posture, though fieldwork suggests that medical students progressively lose sight of this possibility as they seek to establish professional competence. In fact, by the time my research was completed and I had given it more thought, I found that I had moved quite far from my own original position. I learned to distrust the bedside manner, the charming mien of the physician, as a test of competence, for some of the most charming physicians were the least competent. I had also lost faith in the prospect of the "Renaissance" physician, the individual who would combine competence, personality, research ability, and common sense. So in denying idealism, I seemed to be affirming cynicism, or the bankruptcy of optimism.

Contemporary physicians practicing in the research-oriented setting of a university are technicians of a superlative sort. They are well acquainted with the most recent literature, can reflect on a constellation of evaluative techniques unavailable to the local physician, and can exploit the most brilliant minds in specialties outside their own competence. After living among them for many months, I have no reservations about seeking their assistance in the event of a serious medical problem; for I would rather take my chances on the coldest, most detached of clinical investigators than forgo the benefits of their clinical expertise. Now it would appear that I am overlooking the numerous social and psychological variables affecting patient recovery that are intrinsically tied to the doctor-patient relationship, apart from the mastery of technique. This distinction is more than the artifice of argument. Internal to the distinction between primary care and medical specialization is the germ of a division of labor based upon the healer-curer dichotomy espoused by Eric Cassell.[8] Let the primary-care physician or practitioner be the health-care professional with whom I develop a long-term affective relationship nurtured with mutual trust and respect. It is to this person I turn for the preponderance of my medical needs, the self-limiting colds and viruses. This primary-care professional would be responsible for noting the role of my social-psychological needs as they impinge on health care. This person would serve as my initial contact with health-care services and, as the need arose, the source of referral to the specialist as technician. In this fashion, even if my relationship with the specialist is devoid of emotional satisfaction, the primary practitioner serves as a liàison between the two forms of focus. And in the event there is nothing the specialist can do to ameliorate my condition, let me return to my physician-healer, who can share in my anguish as well as admit his or her own discomfort in the absence of anything to do. For the needs of the chronically ill are frequently predicated on psychosocial support, regardless of available clinical options.

I am not saying that healing and curing are necessarily mutually exclusive. I only wish to acknowledge a saddening reality, the absence of *both* Hygeia and Asclepius within medical practice.[9] Once I confront that reality, I can consider the alternatives available to me.

I do not see change coming from physicians, for they have too large a stake in their own survival and the protection of their prerogatives. They deal with anxious, worried people who often deny their illnesses and then blame the physician because he or she can do so little. They labor under their own exaggerated notions of what medicine can do, and when their limitations press against them, they feel discomfort, anger, and exhaustion. Many physicians, in the early stages of their career, seek a role model, someone who will understand their predicament and then transcend it by providing an example of how a physician can be both a human being and a clinician. On the surface this appears to be a peculiar way of posing a problem of limitation, for we all know that physicians are human beings. Yet the normal recreations—athletics, family, social life, the arts—which provide a context for renewing the nonprofessional self are all too often pushed aside as the demands of the role require continuing education in addition to lengthy hours of office practice, hospital rounds, and administrative duties. Professional performance within the highly competitive research setting frequently demands personal depletion. As the personal, private self is overwhelmed by the professional self, it is not difficult to see how the person suffering from nephritis becomes "the diseased kidney." Thus, if one spends enough time with physicians, one can perceive their vulnerability at the same time that one becomes enamored of their privileges.

Both physicians and nonphysicians often see the extravagant financial rewards of medicine as ample reimbursement for personal depletion, or the loss of the aspect of self which exists independent of professional identity. Yet after one reaches a point of significant income, money can be no substitute for time for self and others. Pay alone cannot redeem a profession which leads to a loss of self, or which requires the sacrifice of professional achievement in order to secure the "wholeness" of the individual.

In the many hours and months I spent with medical students and physicians I learned to see both their vulnerabilities and their strengths, to appreciate the intellectual stimulation of medicine, and to lose faith in an assumption of individual responsibility. While I find it impossible to condemn physicians in general for their performance, I am much chastened by what I saw and learned. While there were people whom I learned to admire and respect, there were a good many who did little that was commendable. A few seemed truly reprehensible, though their shortcomings were not founded in personal malice. As I see it, they were trapped in the limitations of their narrow professional lives, so that they could no longer see beyond personal achievement and aggrandizement. Yet as my understanding of their professional socialization increased, so did my empathy. I could become angry, but not bitter. I could see what they had failed to notice.

Almost from the beginning, it was clear that by virtue of my training and experiences I did not share in their reality. It was not that theirs or mine was better—just different. As I followed the second-year student, the third-year student, and the fourth-year student through clinical rotations on medical services, I watched their reality shift, until they came to think of themselves as physicians long before they were awarded their degrees. I listened as attending physicians instructed them on becoming a "good physician," defined as one who is compulsively thorough and who accepts responsibility, and I realized that they did not share in my "lay" definition. I noted a difference between what medical students and their teachers thought to be relevant information in taking a patient's history, and those questions I might have pursued. And somehow they were always surprised when I suggested a question they had overlooked which proved relevant.[10] More important, even as I learned the "clinical material" in the fashion of a second-year student, I had difficulty in restricting my conceptual universe to diseased organs and blood biochemistry. Their attitude toward what they saw and heard led to a narrowing of focus down to its fullest expression, commitment to a medical specialty. In contrast, I, ebullient with this new clinical knowledge, wanted to focus out, to integrate it somehow with my sociological awareness in order to articulate the specialness of clinical thinking.

In subsequent chapters, therefore, the reader will find four major divisions of argument. In the first part of this book I wish to demonstrate that ethical issues abound in the clinical setting, but are rarely framed in terms of any formal ethical analysis. The "clinical mentality," as Eliot Freidson calls it,[11] has rules of right and wrong which determine "acceptable practice," but it is an ethical system that is severely shrunken in scope. In fact, there is a tendency to translate ethical issues into technical problems which have clinical solutions. A series of case histories will demonstrate the visible and invisible facets of these ethical issues. The second part of the book provides a theoretical framework for examining different moral universes based on the clinical, legal, and moral perspective. The third part depicts the professional socialization of medical students during their clinical rotations on medical (as opposed to surgical) services in a university research hospital. It will be argued that there is a gradual falling-off of ethical concern in students' professional behavior and an increasingly strong identification with the clinical perspective, together with a secondary component of the legal perspective. Finally, in the fourth part, some policy considerations are outlined which evolve from the recognition of institutional, role, and personality constraints on physician performance.

In part, this book is an exhortation to the lay public: think about the problematic developments in contemporary medicine before you find yourself facing them as a patient or as a relative of a patient. Physicians are no smarter, no more well versed in the management of these problems of control over living and dying than we who defer to their presumed wisdom. Even when we are powerless to find answers which seem consistent with fairness, with humility, with the enhancement of what it means to be "human," we need to raise the questions, explore our assumptions, evaluate the range of possible answers. The very act of analysis moves us further from the dangers of moral suasion and rhetoric that are founded in fuzzy thinking and emotional hysteria. We seek answers that are consistent with rationality and compassion, and that is a difficult pair of conditions to satisfy.

We demand more of physicians than we have a right to ask of

them, since they are merely human beings like ourselves. We are all too willing to let them assume the total responsibility for confronting these ethical issues, while we stand quick to judge the "rightness" of their actions, devoid of an understanding of how and why they think as they do. And they, with a prideful arrogance, greedily take the responsibility, for it enhances their status in the eyes of the laity and bolsters their authority over a wide range of social concerns. For after all, would many of us who are not physicians wish to make decisions about life and death nearly every day?

What follows is an explication of those differences in moral view which seem to make the grounds for mutual help so elusive. The adversary relations between patients and physicians as reflected in the skyrocketing rates of malpractice insurance are signs of fundamental problems within the medical establishment; their resolution requires a serious rethinking of both medical education and the delivery of health-care services.

PART ONE

Three Cases

1 Getting "Buzzed"

She was a stoop-shouldered old lady whose gray, greasy hair was pushed back with tortoise-shell combs. Her navy plaid jumper was shabby, with buttons missing and the hem held up by safety pins. Her baggy blouse was yellow with age. She wore tan, opaque stockings of an indestructible material; they bagged around thin ankles. She would have seemed at home on Ellis Island. As a new patient in the in-house psychiatric unit, she was described on her chart as "a 77 year old white woman with multiple medical problems focused on her GI [gastrointestinal] system, who came in because she is depressed." Sadie Myers could tell you of the pain in her belly, her poor vision, her diabetes, the excruciating pain in her back and legs, and how she was alone in the world with no one to care whether she lived or died. Her only surviving brother was bedridden with a stroke; when he saw her, he thought she was his mother. She was all alone in a big house, which she said was her whole life since her husband had died two years ago. She described her dead husband as a former subject of the czar, and as a jealous, tyrannical man who was suspicious of people, who kept her tied to their "slavery [grocery] store" for more than forty years. Her whole life has been a tale of misery, unimproved by his death. During the past two years she has become increasingly depressed. Her somatic complaints multiplied, and her daily visits and calls to her physician drove him to hospitalize her, first on a medical service and then in the psychiatric unit.

She came in on a Monday, and Tuesday was the day to discuss patients with the attending Dr. Schmidt, a German of Freudian bias, who impressed all the patients with his good looks and soothing manner of speaking. According to Dr. Schmidt, ECT (electroconvulsive therapy)* is the recommended treatment for involutional melancholia, Sadie Myers's diagnosis. † "I think she should be buzzed.‡ It's pathetic enough . . . that she was not assertive enough to get the hell out of her marriage to a husband who was probably psychotic. All her life she has been some kind of *kvetch*."

The same day she was visited by her referring physician, who walked into her room while the team was making rounds and pulled out all the stops as he delivered a grand performance:

Referring physician: Sadie, how long have I known you? Many years. And you know how concerned I am about you. That's why I had you moved here, so you can have all these doctors help you. How many doctors do you have here right now? Five, and they all care and want to help you. Now I want you to stay and cooperate. I've done all I can do for you, so I have turned to professional help. Your problems are not your belly. Now I want you to be good or I shall have to spank you.

After ten days of hospitalization Dr. Schmidt suggested that Sadie Myers be put on Haldol** "in order to calm her down and make

---

*ECT (EST), electroconvulsive therapy, is done in the surgical recovery room. An anesthesiologist administers short-acting anesthetizing and paralyzing agents. The anesthesiologist breathes for the patient, who cannot do so himself. A small "black box" about the size of a typewriter keyboard, with a setting for voltage and duration of voltage is plugged into the wall. The older method of applying electrodes to both sides of the brain (bilateral placement) is no longer used; instead, electrodes are applied at the temple to the nondominant side of the brain only—to avoid the confusion and disorientation that was common with the bilateral method. A mouthpiece prevents the patient from biting his tongue. The anesthesia must take effect before the paralyzing agent works in order to prevent the patient from experiencing the trauma of paralysis (subjectively experienced as drowning and suffocation), and the paralyzing agent must be given early enough to peak at the time of the shock so that there will be no broken bones. The patient is "buzzed" for 0.6 seconds at 150 volts and awakens within five minutes from the start of the procedure having no memory of the shock. Patients get eight to twelve shock treatments for depression, and up to twenty for schizophrenia.

†Involutional melancholia is a depression associated with the menopause or, more generally (and in this case), with the onset of a particular life event, such as the death of a husband or parent.

‡*Buzzed* suggests something relatively benign, the onomatopeia of a bee or deep slumber, which goes along with the university physician's faith in ECT. Sometimes the staff substitute *zapped,* generally in the case of unwilling candidate for ECT.

**Haldol (haloperidol) is a tranquilizer which, according to the *Physician's Desk Reference* (PDR) should not be used in cases of severe depression. It is recommended for "the management of manifestations of psychotic disorders" (p. 969). The list of her more amenable to ECT. When we talk to her in a few days we'll be able to do what we want." Even with her initial dose doubled and then increased daily by increments of 2 mg, she held out. She refused to call her nephew Irving, a physician in the western part of the state, because it would cost too much, but she was insistent on writing him about her physician's plan for ECT. She knew that he would "hit the ceiling when he heard what they wanted to do with her."

Sadie Myers was told that if she refused ECT, the doctors would have to decide on something else, but the focus of influence remained the same: Sadie must sign for ECT.

For the next two weeks Sadie Myers complained about her numerous problems, accepted the hospital routine, and generally made herself at home. She rejected all attempts at getting her other clothes. She contended that none of her neighbors could find her clothes because everything was locked up, and she refused to tell her next-door neighbor where to find her clothes. After two weeks she allowed a nurse to wash her hair, but she complained it was not as good a job as when her hairdresser did it. Her cousin eventually brought her two dresses, but she refused to wear them.

Daily Sadie Myers was told that she would feel better with "electric treatments." She refused, sometimes saying that she was not strong enough for them. One day she admitted that a patient had come in to visit with her and had told her not to take the treatments. She was asked whose word she was going to take, a patient's and a stranger's or her physician's. At this point she was more ambivalent than obstinate.

Two weeks after the initial attempt to get Mrs. Myers to consent to ECT, and with her regime of Haldol showing little positive effect, Dr. Schmidt declared, "Medicine is through with her, psychiatry will make a last ditch effort to get her to sign. Now she is a social disease, and she is yours, Ellen" (Ellen Smith, the social worker).

During the third week of hospitalization, Sadie Myers slipped and fell while trying to close her window and suffered a hairline break

adverse reactions is extensive, including dry mouth, blurred vision, loss of appetite, impaired liver function, rapid heartbeat, hypertension, and Parkinson-like symptoms. The PDR is a standard reference book that can be found in public libraries. It lists all prescription and nonprescription drugs by function and drug company, provides pictures for identification, and lists restrictions (side effects, toxicities) as well as appropriate usage.

in one rib. With her bruises and new pain she was less desirous of leaving the hospital, though she had made speeches about leaving it once her referring physician returned from vacation (the day she fell).

Her referring physician returned and noted on the chart that she had refused ECT, and he informed her there was nothing more he could do for her. He could no longer give her the kind of daily attention she needed. He recommended placement in a retirement home. Her primary therapist, a fourth-year medical student, had failed to persuade her. Dr. Schmidt had failed to charm her into it. Sadie Myers's cousin by marriage, Morris Shapiro, was recruited to convince her that she could be cured with ECT.

Mr. Shapiro, an energetic eighty-year-old, knew his cousin very well and demonstrated skill at exchanging insult for insult. He said that despite her poor refugee appearance, she had lots of money obtained through thievery and conniving. He was prepared to persuade Sadie with the story of a charming, intellectual cousin of seventy-four who had been cured by ECT of her depression. On the seventeenth day of her hospitalization, he maneuvered Sadie close to signing, though he wanted the start of treatment delayed a few days while Sadie gained a bit of strength. An appointment was arranged for the next day for the formal signing.

The signing was attended by Ellen Smith, the resident, Sadie Myers's therapist, the author, Morris Shapiro, and Sadie Myers. Sadie launched into a list of complaints, including the fact that the physical therapy department would not give her treatments for her legs unless they had her physician's permission. Dick, the resident, promised her she would have her treatments if she would only sign the form that would authorize ECT (see form 1). Morris Shapiro handed her the consent form and showed her where to sign. She complained that she could not see the dotted line. "Sadie, if this were a check for $1,000, you could see where to endorse it," her cousin cajoled her. No one read the form to her or asked whether she had any questions about the procedure. Of course, the mechanics of it had been explained to her many times before. She signed. Morris Shapiro acted as witness, and then he excused the two of them from the office.

The resident, the medical student, and the social worker were satisfied that Sadie Myers had given her informed consent. The nature of the procedure had been explained, and she had been told that the probability of a cure was high, though not certain. She had been

FORM 1

PSYCHIATRIC INPATIENT DEPARTMENT
UNIVERSITY HOSPITAL

Permission for Electroconvulsive Treatment

I hereby request and grant my permission to the doctors of the Psychiatric Inpatient Department of the University to administer electroconvulsive therapy as indicated in the case of ....

I recognize that there may be risks involved and intending to be legally bound do release the doctors, the Hospital and The Trustees of the University Hospital from all liability in connection therewith.

An explanation of this treatment has been given me by Dr. ...., and I am aware of the following circumstances and risks:

A controlled electric current is passed between two electrodes attached to the patient's temple, which stimulates the brain, and produces muscle contractions throughout the body. Danger to life is about the same as the risk of general anesthesia for a surgical procedure. The most frequent complications are occasional fractures and dislocations. Some degree of temporary memory impairment and confusion is frequent: care must therefore be taken, based on the physician's recommendation, as to the time after treatment when business responsibilities and exposure to dangers of traffic, etc., may be resumed.

While results of treatment are usually gratifying, they cannot be precisely predicted, nor can the number of treatments which will be required be predicted in advance.

Anesthetic and muscle-relaxant (Sodium Brevital and/or Anectine) medications may or may not be used, depending on individual conditions which may change during the course of treatment.

I grant the permission and give the release as above stated, and I am aware of the following conditions which increase the probable risk of treatment: ....

....

(If none, write "None")

Signature of patient:

....

Signature of spouse

or relative ....

Witness: How related ....

....   Address ....

Date: ....

advised that she would be evaluated by an anesthesiologist for possible factors of risk. She had agreed in writing to an unspecified number of daily ECT treatments. She was told that treatments would end when she got better, and neither she nor her cousin raised any objections to the indefinite nature of this regimen. It was acknowledged that she had the right to refuse ECT, but she was also told that the service had no obligation to keep her in the hospital once she refused the recommended treatment.

When I asked about the legality of the ECT consent form, the resident told me there was no problem, because informed consent was simply a matter of patient-physician relations. Even a patient who was a lawyer could be convinced to sign the form, whatever its legal flaws, once persuaded of the benefit to be derived from the procedure. Nor was he persuaded that psychiatric patients might be unable to give true "informed consent" because of their impaired mental status, and consequently might need court-appointed guardians to protect their interests. Just as house staff regularly take skull x-rays of patients who have suffered head injuries for "medical-legal" reasons rather than for their diagnostic value, (which is negligible), written consent is obtained for ECT for the sake of satisfying "medical-legal" requirements, without regard to the intended function of informed consent.

Intelligence and reality testing showed that Sadie Myers was capable of understanding the nature of electroconvulsive therapy. At one point she had attempted to coax a cab voucher out of Ellen Smith, the social worker, and when this failed, she spoke to the head of social services. She knew how to work a system for her benefit. Yet her depression was characterized by unassertiveness, passivity, and refusal to take responsibility for herself. It was as if she had been caught in the mesh of life events and could not attempt to untangle herself, lest she have to decide what she could do outside the net. Consequently, it was highly unlikely that she could mobilize her strength to combat the pressures to sign the consent form. She said she continued to live because she did not know how to go about dying. When asked to sign, she said she might as well be dead so it did not matter if the shock treatments killed her; she just did not want to suffer anymore. Her signing was only another aspect of being coerced by those persons stronger than herself, though this ceased to be the language of her explanation once she grew comfortable on the ward.

Sadie Myers could say, "You cannot make me change my

clothes." The staff repeatedly urged her to get her hair done or to go out on pass and buy some clothes, but her refusal gave her some control over the situation. As long as she could waver between refusing and consenting to ECT, she could manipulate the situation to her benefit. Ultimately she could not hold out against the threatened rejection by her physician of long standing, her therapist, and her cousin. Their rallying around her for the sake of securing her signature was a significant event in her vacant life. It meant that some people cared what she did with her remaining years. To say no in the face of that concern was to make her fears of abandonment come true. She capitulated to the command to sign, giving her "optimistic consent," for what did she have to lose?

Aside from the argument that ECT was the most appropriate treatment, Sadie Myers was evaluated as a candidate for ECT because she was being too demanding of the time and patience of her referring physician. While he was concerned with her emotional improvement, as a specialist in diabetes he was not equipped to deal with her psychiatric problems. Once an extensive physical examination and laboratory studies revealed no organic basis for her depression, he fulfilled his obligation to her by referring her to the psychiatric unit. Since something remained to be done for her clinically, it was not incumbent on him to offer his services as a professional handholder.

ECT was offered in the belief that it would do Sadie Myers less harm than good. It could not be guaranteed that she would recover by virtue of these treatments; rather, there was a probability of benefit. Given that she did not have the expertise to evaluate the usefulness of ECT, Sadie Myers had to accept this recommendation as a matter of faith in the competence of her doctors. Thus, the only test of the rightness or wrongness of their recommendation would be the outcome of her experience; she would get better, get worse, or remain the same. If she believed that human beings desire to do good, she would have an easier time accepting their recommendations than if she believed the reverse; but the test of the matter would remain the same either way.

Although the hospital staff believed they were acting in Sadie's best interests, and despite their confidence that they had satisfied the requirements of informed consent, they failed to examine a number of issues.

According to the guidelines for the protection of human subjects issued by the U.S. Department of Health, Education, and

Welfare (HEW), the following information must be given to the patient in order to meet the definition of "informed consent" in activities supported by grants or contracts from the department. These guidelines pertain to the use of human subjects in research settings only; in nonresearch settings they are merely recommendations rather than legal statutes.

1. A fair explanation of the procedures to be followed, and their purposes, including identification of any procedures that are experimental;
2. A description of any attendant discomforts and risks reasonably to be expected;
3. A description of any benefits reasonably to be expected;
4. A disclosure of any appropriate alternative procedures that might be advantageous for the subject;
5. An offer to answer any inquiries concerning the procedures;
6. An instruction that the person is free to withdraw his consent and to discontinue participation in the project or activity at any time without prejudice to the subject.

"No such informed consent, oral or written, . . . shall include any exculpatory language through which the subject is made to waive, or to appear to waive, any of his legal rights, including any release of the organization or its agents from liability or negligence."[1]

An examination of the permission form signed by Sadie Myers (form 1) reveals that the first paragraph violates the prohibition of release from liability. The fifth paragraph contains no provision for informing the patient of a change in medication or for renewing consent. There are also several omissions of consequence. There is no statement of alternative modes of treatment or probable benefit. There is no notice that the patient may withdraw from treatment at any time without penalty. There is no safeguard of the patient's right to ask questions or any operational check on comprehension (for example, a witnessed statement by the informing physician that the patient can state the nature of treatment in his or her own words).

There are numerous questions of validity. What is the meaning of a patient's signature on a consent form when he or she is receiving medications that may be sedating or in other ways interfering with mental and emotional functioning? If without such medication the same patient would refuse to sign, is the signature valid? Can a patient who suffers from real or imagined fears of psychiatric commitment, divorce, or other disruption of social ties ever give "free and informed consent"? Why is the signature of the spouse or a relative required when the patient is not declared legally incompetent? If the relative's signature is valid in lieu of the patient's, this is an informal declaration of incompetence. Can the relative's signature alone be legally binding? If it is needed to support the patient's consent, this raises the question of usurping the patient's right to autonomy, to accept or to reject treatment as she or he sees fit. If the relative is merely acting as a witness, why is there a second place for the signature of a witness?

A strict interpretation of this situation makes light of these violations, for as long as the patient is not an experimental subject in a project funded by HEW, there is little form of redress beyond questioning the hospital administrators. Refusal to sign is simply a rejection of offered treatment; it absolves the hospital of further responsibility.

The consent form has a manifest institutional function as a gauge of patient-physician cooperation and, viewed in this light, its dubious legal validity is of secondary importance to those who use it.[2] In effect, the legal utility of the document becomes its latent function. Throughout the hospital, informed consent is treated as a necessary evil, untenable in clinical practice, though it is necessary to go through the motions. In order to see this more clearly, we must return to the medical aspects of this situation.

The case of Sadie Myers was a rare example of consensus among the referring physician, the psychiatric attending physician, the resident, and the medical student. As far as they were concerned, she was an ideal candidate for ECT. Her age, sex, and diagnosis all made it probable that ECT would help relieve her depression. By their report, a search of the literature as well as clinical experience indicated that this was the appropriate treatment.

Alternative forms of treatment would include antidepressant medications or psychotherapy. The latter depends on the patient's capacity for insight based on verbal modalities of analysis; both require long periods of time for effectiveness. Twelve Webster, the in-house psychiatric unit, considered itself a crisis-intervention center. The average length of stay was between two and three weeks, which was treated as something of a joke, considering that the history and severity of the complaints required more extensive treatment. While follow-up treatment was arranged for all patients before they were discharged, lack of transportation, turnover in therapists, and motivation problems did little to guarantee continuity in therapy. Nevertheless, some patients seemed to benefit from a stay of less than three days in the protected environment of the ward; they were then ready to return home and deal with their problems as best they could. In view of the wish to maximize the probability of a quick cure or marked improvement, it was logical to employ ECT rather than antidepressants or psychotherapy when the patient was an "ideal candidate" for ECT.

The house staff of Twelve Webster offered personal observation as the test of their arguments in favor of ECT. They encouraged patients to talk to other patients who had had ECT and improved. They told of the miraculous cures that had occurred through ECT, though at times it seemed that these stories were told as much for their own persuasion as for the patients'. On Twelve Webster, rejection of ECT as the appropriate therapy for involutional melancholia and other nonendogenous forms of depression was tantamount to rejecting the psychiatrist as truth-teller as well as capable clinician.

Informed consent in such situations is frequently informed coercion and pressured consent. The patient allows himself or herself to be maneuvered into giving consent out of a willingness to conform as a condition of getting better. Patients lack the means of extricating themselves from a situation of apparent kindness and concern. And physicians see no alternative to their role as persuaders and enchanters if they are to offer patients effective treatment. To do otherwise negates their role as physicians. Consequently, the requirements of truly informed consent are rarely fulfilled and stand little chance of being successfully met unless physicians treat the subject seriously, as a tool of medical care, rather than manipulate it to serve their interests.

Physicians believe that patients have an obligation to accept their recommendations for treatment, which are founded in rational arguments and sound clinical practice. Patients must trust their physicians as a condition of the therapeutic enterprise. Consequently, they view informed consent as nothing more than the articulation of this trust. ECT is an excellent example of this concretization of the problems of truth-telling, trust, and responsibility for decisions into a matter of patient trust. When patients responded to the suggestion of ECT with horror and fear, having learned of it through the popular media and the experiences of family members, their physicians were quick to urge them to trust them. The staff associated with Twelve Webster was anxious to convey the painlessness and simplicity of ECT as currently practiced. They disavowed the ECT of the "snakepits."

The discussion so far has failed to make explicit one other aspect of informed consent. The form giving permission for electroconvulsive therapy exemplifies the selection of one specific procedure as requiring informed consent. In reality, numerous other procedures were performed on Sadie Myers that were subsumed by the blanket consent she gave upon admission to the hospital (see form 2). At what point must explicit consent be obtained? Sadie Myers received her daily dose of insulin, and in the latter part of her admission she received Haldol. Her blood was regularly drawn to test for blood-sugar levels. She received x-rays of the chest, spine, and legs. She attended several sessions of physical therapy. Each of these procedures carries risks as well as benefits, yet her consciousness of the risks was not elicited. "Physicians would need secretaries if they were to get informed consent for each invasive procedure," one student argued.* Yet inattention to the problem does not diminish it. The doctrine of implicit consent readily leads to abuse, for it is difficult to see any critical dividing line between situations where implicit trust is warranted and those where explicit questioning of the basis of that trust is vital.

The second set of issues arising out of this vignette focuses on the nature of valid consent as it is derived from medical evaluation of mental function: Who shall decide whether Sadie Myers shall sign for ECT? Can a "crazy" person ever be "informed" of the risks and benefits inherent in procedures recommended by medical professionals or family? Conceivably the decision to accept or reject the recommendation for ECT could be based on the assumed competence of the physician, in conjunction with professional preference, medical literature, and the availability of facilities; but this posture begs the issue of the autonomy of the adult patient.

Generally speaking, we must posit that adults can decide for themselves what they wish to be done with their bodies, unless there are grounds to believe that they will do themselves harm. In this case, the fear that Sadie Myers might do herself harm was derived from her

---

*An invasive procedure is one which creates injury to healthy tissue, such as securing a blood sample. In general, a case is made for informed consent for invasive procedures.

FORM 2

GENERAL CONSENT FORM

All patients admitted to University and affiliated hospitals
must sign this form as a condition
of their admission.

Authorization for Medical or Surgical Treatment

In connection with the admission of .... (herein called
the "Patient") to the University Hospital (herein called the "Hospital"), the
undersigned hereby authorizes, requests and consents to the performance by the
physicians in charge of the Patient, and by other physicians designated by
them, of such diagnostic procedures, anesthesia, operations, and other medical
or surgical treatment as they may believe to be necessary, advisable or
beneficial for the health or well-being of the Patient. The foregoing
authorization, request and consent shall extend and be applicable to the
Hospital and to the nurses, technicians and other persons employed by or
associated with it who may be engaged in the medical or surgical treatment of
the Patient referred to above. No revocation of this authorization shall be
effective unless and until a written notice of such revocation has been delivered
to the administrator of the Hospital and to the physician in charge of the
Patient's care.

Witness: ....
                                     Signature
                                Address: ....
                                ....
Dated: ....   Relationship to Patient:
                                ....

refusal of treatment that had been identified as potentially helpful. But it was not a matter of life or death, so there was no attempt to formalize the need for a guardian. Instead, kinship ties were exploited to achieve the desired end. Sadie Myers had to decide for herself, but she was coached.

In addition to alternative types of therapy, there are alternatives to the handling of informed consent that increase patient autonomy at the expense of physician autonomy. The following alternatives might be considered:

1. A physician other than the treating physician could administer informed consent, providing the patient with necessary information for a decision and evaluating the patient's comprehension of the proposed procedure. This task might fall to someone other than a physician, such as a nurse-practitioner, who could take the time to fulfill the requirements of informed consent. This would enable the patient to ask questions about the procedure without seeming to question the competence or good intentions of the physician; it also removes some of the pressure on the patient to go along with whatever the physician wants.

2. Patients need to be informed of their right to refuse procedures without penalty. They may fear that they will be discharged, that they will receive even less attention from nurses and physicians, that they will be threatened with a loss of privileges (including visitors), or that they will be denied medical services at a later time.

3. Patients need to be informed that they may consult another physician of their choice, and they should be given instructions as to how to go about this. This may entail instruction on how to contact the local medical society to obtain the names of other specialists, or information on how to secure additional information from other
   - hospital or community resources. While the financial burden would fall to the patient, insurance companies might find it in their interest to pick up this charge, if it proves in the long run to save them money. Indeed, Medicare will now pay for second opinions.

4. Patients need to know that their inability to make a decision does not necessarily transfer that decision-making power to the treating physician. They should be encouraged to talk over the decision with family members or friends in nonemergency situations.[3]

5. Upon completion of the history-taking and physical examination at the time of admission, the physician would obtain informed consent

for diagnostic procedures. The standard admissions package could include a formal record of informed consent, which would consist of a check-off sheet of the most common diagnostic procedures and a simple definition of their purpose. It would also inform patients of any discomfort or risk that might be associated with the procedure. On some services it is already common practice to give the patient an informative brochure. The physician would inform the patient that if additional procedures are required, the patient will have the opportunity to question and review the recommendation and to give or to refuse informed consent. This function might also be performed by a nurse-practitioner.

While many physicians informally fulfill the conditions of the fifth recommendation, a formal stipulation would have multiple functions. It would serve the legal function of informed consent. It would promote patient responsibility in the therapeutic enterprise. It would force the physician to acknowledge limitations on his or her autonomy and to accept increased physician-patient interaction. Such focused attention on the patient as a person[4] would probably heighten patient compliance rather than intensify mistrust, though at this time this is only a hypothesis.[5]

Sadie Myers received ten treatments with little positive effect, though her cousin was convinced she was greatly improved. He arranged for her to go to a nursing home until an apartment became available for her at a prestigious "retirement home" run by a religious organization.

In table 1 the clinical, legal, and ethical issues presented by this case are cited, with acknowledgment of the difference between my elaboration of the issues as a sociologist and the physicians' recognition of the relevant issues. Sometimes physicians made some mention of an issue without treating it from a formal perspective. For example, while the attending physician remarked that Sadie Myers was given Haldol in order to make her more compliant, he never addressed that issue from either a legal or an ethical perspective. A limitation of this table and the tables in the next two case studies is that they treat each issue as a discrete problem, while in reality the boundaries of the issues are frequently blurred. Clearly coercion is both a legal and an ethical issue, with a significant degree of overlap.

TABLE 1

Case of Sadie Myers
Electroconvulsive Therapy (ECT) as "Treatment of Choice" for
Involutional Melancholia in a Seventy-seven-year-old Female

Clinical Issues

(1) Diagnosis of involutional melancholia*
(2) Management of additional physical complaints (back pain, belly pain, etc.)*
    (a) establish organicity as origin
    (b) establish psychogenic origin
    (c) establish contribution of aging
(3) Referral of patient to psychiatric unit by internist*
(4) Establish appropriateness of ECT
    (a) as treatment of choice for involutional melancholia*
    (b) as treatment of choice for Sadie Myers*
(5) use of Haldol*

Legal Issues

(1) Legal competence of patient to give informed consent
    (a) psychiatric hospitalization as modifying factor
    (b) fulfillment of voluntariness
(2) Principle of self-determination (right to refuse ECT)
(3) Principle of autonomy in adult patient (availability of other choices)
(4) Satisfaction of informed consent
    (a) description of attendant risks and benefits†
    (b) description of alternative procedures
    (c) offer of additional information or response to questions†
    (d) instruction of right to refuse any or all forms of treatment without penalty as well as the right to discontinue participation at any time.
    (e) indeterminate nature of ECT (no stipulation of number of times of treatment before reevaluation)
    (f) physician use of coercion
        (i)   by other physicians†
        (ii) by support personnel†
        (iii) by use of cousin*
        (iv) by use of medication to increase compliancy†

* Addressed by physicians through stated perspective.
† Addressed by physicians, but not through stated perspective.

TABLE 1
(continued)

Legal **Issues** (cont.)	(v) by threats of termination of patient-physician relationship† (vi) by overselling value of ECT

Ethical
Issues
	(1) Right of physicians to determine the conditions under which a patient will be treated as a mature adult
	(2) Right of physicians to obtain patient compliance through misrepresentation of facts and relationships†
	(3) Physicians as accomplices in naming the nature and conditions of treatment†
	   (a) intimidation through recruitment of other professionals and relatives in order to assert the strength of numbers, e.g., "All these doctors want to help you" you"
	   (c) intimidation through infantilism, e.g., treating the patient as "a bad girl" who ought to be spanked
	   (d) intimidation through hospitalization on a psychiatric service (as opposed to a psychiatric consultation on the medical service)
	   (e) intimidation through medication (Haldol)†

* Addressed by physicians through stated perspective.
† Addressed by physicians, but not through stated perspective.

In the case of Sadie Myers the clinical perspective dominated, though there was some superficial concern with the legal perspective. The ethical perspective was neglected, though the table enumerates the three perspectives as they might have been discussed.

For the house staff of Twelve Webster, "getting buzzed" is a form of therapy which scarcely merits discussion, though in other professional settings this might not be the case. When the fourth-year medical student left the service to complete his psychiatric rotation in another hospital in the university consortium, he was to find that no one at City Hospital favored ECT for the treatment of depression. It was an important lesson for him, by his own report, and worth thinking about in the light of the next case.

2 Being Female

She was an obese child, and large for her age, with a Dutch-boy haircut that emphasized the roundness of her face. She had a flattened nose and narrow blue eyes which darted to her mother and then back to the shaggy-haired doctor with his shirttail pulling out of his trousers. She demanded to know his name and said it haltingly; she became increasingly excited with each of her attempts to recall his name.

The admission schedule posted by the nurses' station listed "Joan Spoon, cardiac catheterization." Cardiac catheterization is used to diagnose and evaluate congenital, rheumatic, and other coronary artery pathology. A catheter, or tube, is passed through a major blood vessel into the heart. Among other things it allows the sampling of blood from specific locations within the heart in order to determine levels of oxygenation. Pressures can be measured within the heart's chambers or great vessels, and contrast material can be injected to evaluate structural defects. The progression of the catheter as well as the pathway of the contrast material can be viewed on a filmstrip, called a *ciné*. While the cardiac catheterization is no longer considered an experimental procedure, there is always the danger of puncturing the walls of the heart or a blood vessel with the catheter.

Joan's admitting physician, Ralph Hodge, was not well liked by the team. They considered him "a gate," someone who admits too many patients who are not really sick for the sake of collecting his fees.

Joan Spoon was an eleven-year-old white female with Down's Syndrome,* two months past menarche. A large percentage of

*Down's Syndrome, also known as Mongolism, is a type of mental retardation associated with a variety of abnormalities, including a flat, pushed-in face with short

32

Down's Syndrome children have structural heart defects, which make them cardiac cripples and poor surgical risks.[1] The cardiac catheterization was being done to see whether her heart could withstand the stresses of a hysterectomy, surgical removal of the uterus.

Alan Latrobe, the third-year medical student who was caring for Joan, hunted down Ralph Hodge for an explanation of her hospitalization. Dr. Hodge admitted, "It's a long drive on a short punt." When pressed to elaborate, he said given her mental deficiency, he was not too concerned about the risk, though he knew that he had to consider it. But it had been 5 P.M. when he had seen the parents at his office, and he had to "fish or cut bait." He had told them to have their local physician draw some blood gases, but he was unable to obtain them because of Joan's inability to cooperate and her "poor" veins.* Ralph Hodge had tried and failed. He decided to go ahead with the admission for catheterization. Alan asked him if he had explained the risks to the parents. Dr. Hodge replied that he had minimized the risk rather than refusing to do the procedure, because "it turns people off, and they go elsewhere to get it done."

John Smythe, a British resident, commented, "It's strange medicine you practice in this country." He was against the idea of a hysterectomy. He thought birth control pills might be the appropriate contraceptive, with the mother administering them each day. Alan thought the risk of side-effects from birth control pills was too high, but John argued that considering the life expectancy of Mongoloids (twenty-two to twenty-five years), Joan would die before the risk became an issue. Smythe thought Dr. Hodge was money-hungry, and the catheterization was easy money. He argued that a tubal ligation at sixteen was a real possibility, but not a hysterectomy at eleven. "After all," he exclaimed, "who is going to rape an eleven-year-old Mongoloid in a protected home environment?"[2]

nose, transverse palmar crease, stubby fingers, broad hands and feet, and laxness of joint ligaments ("double-jointed"). No single sign is diagnostic, and most signs are found in some normal people. Most commonly, the condition is associated with trisomy-21, a genetic mistake in which there are three alleles on the twenty-first gene, as designated in a karyotype.

*Arterial and venous blood gases are useful for evaluating the amount of carbon dioxide and oxygen in the blood and contribute to the understanding of cardiac and pulmonary function. It is a more painful procedure than the routine venipuncture for red- and white-cell counts. If a person has small, fragile ("poor") veins it increases the difficulty of securing a sample on the first try.

Discussion among the attending physicians, interns, and Alan represented divergent views and varying responses:

David Goldstein, attending physician: I wouldn't do the hysterectomy.

John Barry, visiting attending physician: I would.

Paul Silvers, intern: It's not the parents' decision.

John Barry: I would ask for it but we'd have to get the court's permission.

David Goldstein: It should go through the review board.

Alan Latrobe, third-year medical student: Is it going to be done at University Hospital?

David Goldstein: What would you do with a person with a low I.Q. who is not toilet trained? Do you take out his bowels? . . . I'll ask Oscar Fine [referring physician] in private sometime.

After rounds* Dr. Goldstein took John Smythe aside and told him that the risk of catheterization was great, that Joan stood more risk of dying on the table in the catheter lab than during the hysterectomy. "The parents are concerned about their daughter. It is an unnecessary procedure. Why don't you contact Fine and precipitate it by saying 'the house staff is disturbed.' " The call was never made. Neither John Smythe nor anyone else was willing to incur the probable wrath of Dr. Fine, who would resist any criticism of his clinical judgment. The proposed phone call would be a violation of professional etiquette.

Since nothing was done to stop the scheduled catheterization, it was performed. To everyone's surprise, it revealed severe pulmonary hypertension and ventricular septal defect (VSD), two conditions which made Joan Spoon a poor candidate for any kind of major surgery. For the nonphysician it is often difficult to realize that physi-

---

*There are three kinds of regularly scheduled rounds: work rounds, attending (teaching) rounds, and grand rounds. Work rounds occur first thing in the morning on medical services. The team goes around and sees each patient, notes lab tests, bloods, consultations, x-rays, and the like, and picks up any changes in the patient's behavior. Attending rounds generally occur four times a week. The attending physician reviews difficult cases at length with the team, teaches about diagnosis and management of specific diseases, and tries to maintain general familiarity with all the patients on the service. Grand rounds occur once a week for an hour and are attending rounds on a grand scale. One or more patients is presented to the house. The cases that are selected for grand rounds often border on the esoteric.

cians have nothing more than probability in their favor when they claim to know the outcome of a procedure in advance. The mature physician is capable of genuine humility because she or he knows that there is no "sure thing" in medicine. Anticipated disasters fail to materialize, while straightforward cases become difficult emergencies. When Dr. Hodge was asked whether this would change his plans, he characterized the new diagnosis as "a big wrinkle." He admitted there were alternatives to surgery but concluded, "Surgery is not ruled out."

Meanwhile Dr. Goldstein, chairman of the Patients' Rights Committee for Children's Hospital and attending physician for "Older Children's Medical" for a four-week period, pondered the course to take. John Smythe and Alan Latrobe wanted to know what he thought could be done. In the course of the discussion, Dr. Goldstein offered me some time during attending rounds to raise the various legal issues at stake.[3] While the relevant cases were based on the rights of institutionalized mental defectives, the burden of the arguments supported a case against the sterilization of Joan Spoon.

Eight states permit voluntary sterilization of mentally deficient individuals by statute. However, these statutes apply to "adults" as defined by the relevant statute.[4] The Department of Health, Education, and Welfare outlines a general policy stating that programs receiving funds from the federal government

> shall not perform nor arrange for the performance of any non-emergency sterilization unless such sterilization is performed pursuant to a voluntary request for such services made by the person on whom the sterilization is to be performed or by his or her representative.[5]

Using this guideline, the grounds for the sterilization of Joan Spoon collapse into parental convenience.

However, HEW guidelines have been invalidated on the grounds that the mentally incompetent cannot meet the "voluntariness" standard. In *Robinson* v. *California,* the court cited the principle of equal protection of the laws and argued that the mentally defective cannot be subjected to sterilization by virtue of their mental disorder or defect.[6]

Relf v. *Weinberger* provides safeguards against the abuse of power by an institutionalized patient's "representative." It requires review by the hospital review committee as well as by a state court to determine whether the proposed sterilization is in the best interest of the patient.[7] Since the consent of the mental defective is not required, and since the definition of "representative" goes undefined, there is the possibility of arbitrariness in accepting the unexamined work of the representative which this ruling seeks to prevent.

Compulsory sterilization of institutionalized persons can also be construed as cruel and unusual punishment, in violation of the Eighth Amendment. Decisions subsequent to the 1927 case *Buck* v. *Bell*[8] required substantive demonstration of the need to violate the personal right of reproduction;[9] this is in addition to any arguments demonstrating the legitimacy of state interests in the sterilization. Hence, the court must show that there are no viable alternatives to sterilization that would also preclude the progeny of the defective person from becoming a burden on the state.

Finally, if institutionalized individuals are to be deprived of their rights, assuming that sterilization is within the powers of the state, the procedure must comply with the due process clause of the Fourteenth Amendment. Thus, a person subject to a sterilization order should be given a hearing, receive reasonable notice of the hearing, and have the right to counsel (appointed, if indigent), the right to confront witnesses against him or her, have the right to cross-examine witnesses, and the right to offer evidence, including the testimony of medical experts. In the case of incompetents, a guardian should be appointed by the court and receive notice of the hearing.

Thus, on legal grounds there is little to sustain the request for sterilization of Joan Spoon, though it is ironic that as a noninstitutionalized patient Joan Spoon is ensured of less protection of her rights than a patient in a state institution. As a private patient and as a dependent of loving, middle-class parents, she may have suffered because they could institute limiting care without exposing themselves to a challenge of their authority by house officers. They were further insulated by both the referring and admitting physicians, who had their own interests to maintain. If Joan had been institutionalized because of her parents' poverty or neglect, she might have been protected against such violation. If she were poor and black, and her case came into the public eye, it might have constituted a *cause célèbre*. This case illustrates a possible refutation of the standard model of egregious discrimination. The documented violations of legal and moral principles are not just promulgated on the part of physicians against members of minority groups or those who, for any reason, are in a position of powerlessness. They affect all patients, for reasons that go beyond ignorance or callousness.

From the perspective of the protection of physicians' and parental integrity, Dr. Goldstein advised that the parents be told that surgery was not recommended for medical reasons. Joan's heart condition allowed the sidestepping of ethical concerns in favor of sound clinical reasons against surgery. To reveal that there were legal questions at stake would imply that the parents as well as the physicians might be acting improperly; obviously, this would not serve patient-physician relations.

This case is useful because it illustrates how ethical and legal concerns can be collapsed into the clinical perspective. Even though this case provided one of the few opportunities for discussion of ethical and legal issues, it was not at great variance with the predominant schema—the ascendancy of the clinical perspective. If Joan had not had severe pulmonary hypertension, there might have been greater critical importance in the recognition of legal issues. It was also one of the few times I was asked to respond to a problem as a sociologist, and the only time I did so in a formal setting. From time to time I was asked "as a sociologist" what I would advise, but this was the only occasion when I was asked to make a formal presentation during attending rounds. It was also one of the clearest instances of disapproval by doctors of professional behavior. Undoubtedly this was abetted by Dr. Goldstein's position as chairman of the Patients' Rights Committee and by John Smythe's cultural dislocation. A native of the United Kingdom, Smythe was attending Children's Hospital on a postgraduate fellowship. By virtue of his socialization to the norms of Great Britain, he was sensitized to violation of "his norms" within the American cultural milieu. The incongruity between the two normative systems required greater explanation, because of the extensive overlap. If the systems had been acknowledged as radically different, the need for explanation would have been less apparent because it could be accounted for by citing this difference. In fact, of all the physicians I encountered, the ones who stand out by virtue of their formal remarks about ethics were both foreigners. While only a hypothesis, it appears that foreign-born physicians retain the ethical perspective in situations where their American peers lose it because of cultural dislocation, transience (they have no long-term obligations to the host institution, so they need not collapse "ethics" into professional etiquette), and less reliance on technology. Because many foreign physicians expect to return to countries where the practice of medicine is less imbued with a technological ethos, they have to place greater reliance on personal judgment than on technology. Consequently, they are less hesitant to use a moral perspective.

The various clinical, legal, and ethical issues appearing in the case of Joan Spoon are summarized in table 2. In this case the inadvertent message was, Why are we getting so excited when there is nothing we can do? Nobody was willing to challenge the referring physician. Since surgery was scheduled for University Hospital rather than Children's, and since the authority of the Patients' Rights Committee did not extend down the street, there was no way to confront the culpable staff members or guarantee "the right to reproduce" to this child. Instead, the legal and ethical issues were collapsed into the clinical perspective. No surgery was recommended.

This case also illustrates that while students, such as Alan Latrobe, may initiate discussion of ethical issues, it is the prerogative of senior ranking staff to sustain or to extinguish discussion as they see fit. If students raise questions and repeatedly find them ignored or minimized, they cease to risk rebuff. For example, second-year students during their first clinical rotation will ask "What happened to Mr. Jones?" and mean "How did Mr. Jones die?" When they regularly get a succinct answer devoid of ethical connotations "He died at about seven this morning" they learn not to ask about how he was treated in his dying. They would mention to me, "Did you see how they treated her?" The third-year student asks, "Did you see how he treated me?" after the resident gives him a hard time. After a while the medical student stops asking why, he learns to explain for his own satisfaction, "This is what we do." This will be elaborated on in chapter 8. The invisibility of ethical issues is supported by the absence of questions.

Another message of this case is that ethics is a matter of private and unexamined professional behavior unless institutional reasons expose them to general purview. As much as members of the pediatric service were scornful of Ralph Hodge's pursuit of fees, as much as they questioned his clinical judgment, what he did was a matter between him and his patients. If patients found him distasteful, they could go elsewhere. By coincidence, there were people on the medical

TABLE 2

Case of Joan Spoon:
Sterilization of an Eleven-year-old Female
Down's Syndrome Patient

Clinical Issues

(1) Ability of patient to withstand risks of cardiac catheterization*

(2) Significance of mental deficiency in surgical control of reproduction in postmenarche female*

(3) Diagnosis of severe pulmonary hypertension and VSD*

(4) Parents' initiation of request for sterilization (hysterectomy) of daughter*

Legal Issues

(1) Status of patient as it pertains to her inability to give informed consent for herself:
   (a) a minor
   (b) mentally deficient with medical designation of Down's Syndrome
   (c) noninstitutionalized patient

(2) Relevant legal rights which would be infringed upon in the event of sterilization:
   (a) Right to reproduce
   (b) Right to privacy
   (c) Right to self-integrity

(3) Necessity of review of case by ethics committee of hospital where sterilization is to be performed*

(4) Liability of University Hospital for negligence and/or malpractice of physician who subjects patient to unnecessary risks of cardiac catheterization as prerequisite for "unlawful" surgery

(5) Validity of informed consent forms used by University and affiliated hospitals

Ethical Issues

(1) Right of parents to determine reproductive capacity of minor daughter*

(2) Right of physicians to support parents in decision of dubious ethical validity

(3) Physicians as accomplices in the nonprofessional behavior of a colleague

(4) Violation of truth-telling in explanation of risks and benefits of therapy*

*Addressed by physicians through stated perspective.

team for that four-week period who were willing to admit and to address the questionable aspects of his behavior; but they could easily have shut their eyes and their mouths, if only because of his status as a private physician. Everyone within the hospital system knows that if you irritate a private physician too often or push him too far, he is likely to stop referring patients to your service, and empty beds are no way to run a hospital. This is not of particular salience to medical students, who are unpaid labor, but house officers know where their paychecks come from.

So far we have assumed the perspective of the physicians and students who were involved in the case of Joan Spoon. Going past that perspective, we need to raise some additional questions. For one thing, I as a sociologist was asked to delve into the legal issues; there was no mention of the moral issues. This is tantamount to treating the problem as concrete and circumscribed rather than as abstract and diffuse. It is a matter of knowing where to look for codified information that is rational in structure and universally applicable within this system. As a physician, one learns to ask what can realistically be done within existing structures, without questioning those limits. Even though discussion revealed that existing mechanisms of review were inadequate, no one got excited about reform. This is not very surprising, for the further along medical students travel in the course of professional socialization, the more they learn to accept rather than to challenge, despite exhortations by the teaching faculty to question everything. More specifically, students learn to select carefully the arenas for battle so that the chances for being correct are enhanced. In order to maintain one's equanimity amid the normal irritations of bureaucratic life, one learns to treat boundaries as a source of comfort; they mark the domains where one can exist in relative safety. Only the neophyte bangs his head against a stone wall in an attempt to remove the limitation.

Without the issue of mental incompetence, the question of sterilization would not have been raised. One source of Joan's incompetence was her status as a minor. Adult status is generally a basis for consent, though it has been challenged in other contexts. The exceptions include treatment of venereal diseases, procurement of contraceptives, and consent for organ donations to a sibling. The prima facie reason was her I.Q., in the range of 50 to 80 on the Stanford-Binet scale. The more general question is, What defines mental impairment as a limiting factor in patient voluntariness? Under what conditions can the patient accept responsibility for his or her treatment, when informed of the balance of risks and benefits at an appropriate level of communication? The capacity to give consent may vary with such subjective variables as stress, depression, or anger, but it is also a function of some objectively determinable variables: (1) Is mental impairment a function of medical designation, even when the label is not a disease entity, such as "minimal brain dysfunction" or Down's Syndrome? (2) Is it a function of age, leading us to exclude the very young and the very old from the population of "voluntary" patients? (3) Is it a function of education, which is covertly an indicator of social class, such that those with less than an eighth-grade education are de facto "mentally defective"? (4) Is it a function of intellect, so that those with an I.Q. of less than 80 are not capable of giving consent? (5) Finally, is it a function of professional status, given that patients who are lawyers and physicians (or have such professionals within their immediate kinship circles) may be able to influence the granting or withholding of the label of "mentally defective," while those who are truck drivers or unemployed may contribute nothing? Beyond the issue of consent is the issue of basic human rights. Are we suggesting that Joan Spoon may never reproduce because of a genetic defect? Because she is a child? Because she is uneducated or dull-witted? Because she cannot deal with her "guardians" on their level of function? The selection of any one of these characteristics fails to discriminate among the competing issues; for there are other members of these sectors of the population who are not subject to reproductive restriction through sterilization.

Both this case and that of Sadie Myers illustrate the transformation of social problems into medical problems, with the change in the locus of the problem and the increase in the authority of the physician. The increasing transformation of social problems into medical problems has expanded the authority of physicians and extended their power to areas of social life that were once the concern of the clergy and the police. For example, Sadie Myers was not held responsible for her depression as she might have been in a previous era. Joan Spoon is no longer regarded as a sign of God's displeasure with her parents. While such social problems as alcoholism and insanity were once criminal offenses as well as a cause for religious damnation, they have become medical problems requiring the assistance of the physician, who serves as both judge and healer. When social differences become the basis of medical consultation leading to an evaluation of defectiveness, physicians further enrich their roles as judges and healers. The "antisocial" characteristics of the hyperactive child become subsumed under the medical label "minimal brain dysfunction." Mood swings which may reflect social discomfort become medicalized into subcategories of depression. With the medicalization of social life, which in itself fosters passivity and dependency on physicians, we find the abnegation of an ethic of responsibility on the part of patients. This dependency enhances the power of physicians as diagnosticians (evaluators) and technicians (healers).

The cases of Sadie Myers and Joan Spoon differ markedly in their focus on ethical issues: the second case establishes the recognition of ethical issues in the clinical setting. The process by which the ethical issues were brought to the fore is of particular interest because it characterizes situations that will later be described as anomalous— the overt treatment of ethical issues by physicians in University Hospital.

3 Letting Go

Louise Marks never spoke to me. By the time I had arrived in the Medical Intensive Care Unit (MICU) she was beyond words, though she could still squeeze a hand or blink her eyes when instructed to do so. Even though she was sixty-eight it was clear that she had once been a beautiful woman. Toffee-colored hair framed her face in curls. She was of slender build, though her appearance was limited to what was exposed above the sheet. There was no clinical introduction to her dying that made her ''an interesting case'' to the physician and the student.[1] Rather, it was the social description that placed her in my notes.

It was said that she had been an opera star, a soprano, when she was young. She had married well and lived a happy life with a devoted husband. His death two years ago had thrown her into a deep depression. As she ceased to care about her physical needs, her son had arranged for nursing-home placement because the daughter-in-law refused to have the old woman in her home. From then on, Mrs. Marks had become increasingly burdened by her heart condition.

The house staff debated whether she should receive a permanent pacing wire or whether the temporary wire should be pulled in order to see how she would do. If her heart could beat without assistance, she would be sent to the floor. ''Sending a patient to the floor'' is sometimes an informal means of controlling an unpleasant situation. Since there is a lower nurse to patient ratio on a general medical service than in the intensive care unit, patients who are moved to the floor may get less frequent attention. In situations where slowness to act may contribute to death, and where death is desirable, as in the case of the acutely senile patient, the staff will try to send a patient to the floor as quickly as possible.

For example, Andy White, an 80-year-old black man, suffered

43

from cardiac insufficiency. He was so senile that he could do nothing for himself. He would forget he was eating, and keep a mouthful of scrambled eggs in his mouth for hours. The MICU staff was eager to send him to the floor, but difficulty in regulating his medication kept him in the intensive care unit, despite two tries to send him out. Similarly, troublesome patients are sent out faster than "delightful" patients. Dorothy Buzzy was brought into the MICU in a state of respiratory failure. Once she began to show improvement she also created a reputation for herself as "a pain." Both nurses and physicians would report that she purposely urinated in the bed rather than use the bedpan. There was much interest in sending her to the floor as quickly as possible, despite the fact that there were few patients in the MICU.

Finally, the typical patient who comes in off the street will be sent out faster than "a political admission" with the same medical problem. "Political admissions" are prestigious individuals, such as state supreme court justices, who have influential physicians as their private attending physicians. Thus, Emil Astor, a wealthy corporation president, stayed in the MICU longer than the routine stay for post-surgical complications because his private physician insisted that he needed the round-the-clock nursing of the MICU. Despite his affluence, no move was made to suggest he personally employ a private-duty nurse.

Fatolah Paz, the resident, thought that Louise Marks's wire should be pulled, in order not to prolong her "d/cing" (dying). Arnold Jones, one of the two interns, agreed. When Arthur Gold, an eminent cardiologist, came in for attending rounds, he was polled for his opinion:

Dr. Gold: If she's mentally incapable of profiting from a permanent pacemaker, I see no reason for putting it in. The profession tends to overtreatment. In this case we have made a decision not to press pharmacological therapy.

Since Arthur Gold was respected by the house staff, despite his displays of self-importance, his opinion mobilized them. Paz asked Arnold Jones to speak to the house staff on Walker 8, the general medical service, as well as to the attending physician on that service. Furthermore, the private physician had to be told of the plan to inform everyone involved in her care that she was a "no code." An emergency call for all available staff is called a "code" or a "stat" (short for *statim,* immediately). Next to each bed in the MICU there is a red emergency button which sounds an alarm. When a code is called, anyone who hears it dashes to the site of the emergency, for during the first few minutes extra hands are urgently needed. Generally one person takes charge, usually a resident, and calls out directions to others in the room. A "no code" is simply a situation where the alarm will not be sounded in the event of a life-threatening emergency.

This had to be done before Mrs. Marks left the unit, because anyone who was responsible for the house and was unaware of her status would do the responsible thing of "putting in a wire" in order to save her. The "law of strangers" requires that a physician who comes upon or is presented with a patient about whom he or she knows nothing is required to mount an extensive effort to resuscitate the patient. In this situation, the doctor is not to question whether it might be in the interest of the patient to die, as is the case where the caring physician is familiar with the patient's situation and knows, for example, that the patient is suffering from end-stage cancer. Every senior physician can tell a story about getting burned by upholding this law. Dr. Gold advised that he thought it reasonable to pull the wire and wait to see what happened.

Two days later Louise Marks was still in the MICU, as communication was not yet complete with the medical service that was to receive her. At one o'clock that afternoon she went into "v-tach" and "v-fib," and it was picked up on the monitor at the nurses' station.* Alice, the nurse, got Fatolah Paz, who came into the room and gave Louise one thump on the chest and then a second. (A "thump" is external cardiac massage; the physician bangs on the breast bone to compress the heart and maintain circulation.) Alice reminded him that Mrs. Marks was a "no code." Paz acknowledged that she was a "no thump" and a "no code," but he had forgotten about it in his automatic response to the situation. He did not think that this crisis would mean permanent brain damage if she came out of it. He gave her some

---

*V-tach (ventricular tachychardia) is an abnormally fast heartbeat (rates greater than 100 per minute) originated in an abnormal site. V-fib (ventricular fibrillation) is abnormally rapid contraction of the ventricular muscle that replaces normal contraction of the upper chambers of the heart. If these conditions cannot be brought under control, they are preliminary to cardiac death.

xylocaine* and had Alice give her another injection, but her heart continued in its erratic rhythm. Paz walked over and pulled off Mrs. Marks's oxygen mask. Alice sighed, "She's happier now."

We stood beside her bed and watched her become cyanotic. We stared at the bedside monitor. Paz asked Dick Olson, the other intern, to call her private physician. The latter sent back his thanks for her care and agreed to call her son, because he had some rapport with him. For nearly twenty minutes Arnold and Dick and a nurse stood and stared at the screen, watching the process of death. Finally Roberta, one of the nurses, called from the floor monitor, "Arnold, you have a flat wave now,"[2] and Mrs. Marks was officially pronounced dead by Arnold Jones.

When I first spoke with Dick Olson about the presence of ethical issues in medicine, he contended that ethical attitudes are shaped before medical school. He claimed that no practicing physician worries about ethical issues as a means of clarifying patient management: "You don't sit around worrying whether you should have done this or that in light of moral issues. You do what you can do, and when you can do no more, you stop." What he and others were to express in their words and actions was the enactment of a simple principle: energies should be directed to the living. The moral perspective is implicit in this formulation, for it is the living who can most benefit from the physician's actions. The point at which a person becomes "dead" was irrelevant, by their standards.

During the rest of the month five other patients died. They did not all receive the same degree of extensive medical support, and no matter how pressed, each person involved in their care contended that decisions were made on clinical grounds. Sometimes a patient slipped from "salvageable" to "nonsalvageable" and back to "salvageable" before death claimed him.[3] And at times it appeared that energy was being expended for no purpose other than to give the fourth-year student experience. No one ever admitted that a person could have a "right to die," because there was no room for such a notion within their perspective; yet they did distinguish between patients who had greater and lesser degrees of "social death" prior to their actual de-

---

*Xylocaine hydrochloride (lidocaine hydrochloride) is given intravenously for the management of ventricular arrythmias that occur during surgery, for example, and for life-threatening arrhythmias.

mise. In any case, the social reality was always converted into clinical terms.

While there were no articulated criteria, the house staff distinguished between socially active and socially declining patients, between those who were actively enmeshed in strong family networks and those who were being abandoned by their families. They also maintained a less active stance toward those with impaired brain function, such as the demented patient. They were less inclined to work hard on patients with a history of long-term alcohol or cigarette abuse than on patients hospitalized because of sudden, acute crises. Few physicians favored overly aggressive action on behalf of patients seventy or over unless they were exceptionally healthy and active—still doing physical labor, climbing mountains, and so on. Whether you call it a latent calculus of social worth or simply a matter of utilitarian efficacy, physicians differentiate among patients in terms of their probable salvageability with reference to nonclinical criteria, though some physicians give such factors as social death more weight than others.

The "right to die" is a peculiar claim that has arisen with the growth of medical technology.[4] On the one hand, it is a claim to the right of control over one's dying; on the other, it is an admission that one has no more control over one's dying than over the other events of one's life. It is an argument that one can live too long and grow too weary to find meaning in existence. The problem is, To whom is this right addressed: to the family, to the physician, or to the priest? And what can any of them do in response to the request? The literature on euthanasia is extensive.[5] It pretends to concrete proposals of ethical redress for human misery, but it fails to place the issues in the clinical setting in which they arise. And, as demonstrated in the case of Louise Marks's death, nothing is done in medicine on isolated grounds of ethicality, despite the realness of the question, What is to be gained by continuing this life when mental function is impaired?

The so-called right to die has three subordinate arguments. First, physicians may allow patients to die by acts of medical omission when mental impairment is irremediable.[6] Second, patients or their representatives may instruct physicians to limit medical care to the relief of suffering as a condition of their dying.[7] Third, the assumption is made that "life for life's sake" is not a sufficient reason for committing medical resources to the sustenance of life. The first argument rests on a distinction between active and passive measures that precipitate death, with the latter not identified with euthanasia. The omission-commission argument rests on "proximate cause": did the action or inaction cause the death or merely contribute to its occurrence. For example, you see a child drowning in a pond. You fail to try to rescue the child. Have you killed the child? No, but you did contribute to that child's death. I think the distinction is meaningless in terms of assigning culpability or providing moral guidance. In a clinical setting, no one asks whether pulling the plug is an act of commission or omission, for in the decision to pull the plug the judgment has already been made that the patient is in an irreversible condition of moribundity.

The second argument demands that the "Living Will" (form 3) or its equivalent, though not legally binding, requires respect, even if the physician believes that the patient can surmount the immediate crisis. Among physicians such a document is of little value because of its "Catch-22": If the document was executed and signed during a period of well-being, then it was signed during a time when the person could not realistically evaluate his or her desires in a condition of moribundity. If the document was executed and signed during a period of illness and incapacitation, then it was signed under the duress of incapacity, when physical and mental impairment may have contributed to the decision to sign. In either case, the document is of questionable validity.

The third argument requires that the physician draw limits on his commitment to resuscitation, lest a snowball effect occur; that is, the more time, energy, and material resources invested in the patient, the more likely it becomes that additional resources will be committed to the battle against death.

While there have been court decisions establishing the patient's right to refuse treatment, the underlying principle has been compatible with clinical argument.[8] That is, patients do not have a right to refuse treatment when there are reasonable grounds to believe that treatment will return the patient to an acceptable level of functioning; where the treatment is only a means of "buying time," however, patients have been supported in their claim.[9]

From a legal standpoint, the right to die has generally been converted to other claims that are more readily recognized as legally conferred rights, such as the "right to self-integrity"[10] or "the right to

FORM 3

LIVING WILL

TO MY FAMILY, MY PHYSICIAN, MY LAWYER, MY
    CLERGYMAN
TO ANY MEDICAL FACILITY IN WHOSE CARE I HAPPEN TO BE
TO ANY INDIVIDUAL WHO MAY BECOME RESPONSIBLE FOR
    MY HEALTH, WELFARE OR AFFAIRS

Death is as much a reality as birth, growth, maturity and old age—it is the one certainty of life. If the time comes when I, ..., can no longer take part in decisions for my own future, let this statement stand as an expression of my wishes, while I am still of sound mind.

If the situation should arise in which there is no reasonable expectation of my recovery from physical or mental disability, I request that I be allowed to die and not be kept alive by artificial means of "heroic measures." I do not fear death itself as much as the indignities of deterioration, dependence, and hopeless pain. I, therefore, ask that medication be mercifully administered to me to alleviate suffering even though this may hasten the moment of death.

This request is made after careful consideration. I hope you who care for me will be morally bound to follow its mandate. I recognize that this appears to place a heavy responsibility on you, but it is with the intention of relieving you of such responsibility and of placing it upon myself in accordance with my strong convictions, that this statement is made.

Date ....   Signed ....

Witness ....   Witness ....

Copies of this request have been given to:

....

....

privacy.''[11] When the right to die is conceptualized as a claim to compensation of injury which asks death as its award, then the argument slips into a form modeled after the ''wrongful life'' argument. This arose from cases of illegitimate children who petitioned the court for damages acquired through their bastard status, claiming that they would be better off dead.[12] The courts responded that if the child had not been born, there would have been no mechanism for a tort, since damages can only be awarded to persons, recognized as such through birth.[13] Thus, if the courts were to recognize a claim to ''wrongful life,'' it would also be the condition of extinguishing the basis for ''rights,'' dependent upon ''personhood.''

In considering the professional role of the physician, we must address the limits of medicine to effect change for the better in the patient.[14] In a sociological context this means the patient's recovery to social behavior.[15] A definition that rests on a return to body function is frequently impossible, while a person may be restored to a system of social relations even though he or she suffers from gross body impairment. Thus, palliative measures can be meaningful in the context of returning the patient to a normal environment, which entails the possibility of social relations. As long as the patient remains defined as ''a person'' as opposed to a ''vegetative body,'' he or she will receive aggressive attention. That is, a patient who is strong enough, sufficiently communicative, and a member of a caring family unit will be recognized as a person and will be treated optimistically and aggressively to sustain life. A patient who is strong enough to make a claim to a right to die is also a patient who fulfills a definition of personhood, so there is little likelihood that the claim will be respected, unless there are strong clinical grounds to define an irremediable condition. For example, among physicians in medical (as opposed to surgical) specialities, it is commonly admitted that cancer of the esophagus is a horrible way to die; a patient with cancer of the esophagus may be granted minimal support regardless of whether there is any articulated claim to a right to die. In general however, the only patient who is recognized as having a right to die is one whose premorbid state is so severe that he is without the capacity for social relation, including the ability to communicate ''I don't want to live,'' except in the silent disengagement from all surrounding activity. Consequently, the idea that patients have a right to die is an anomaly within the logic of medicine. For the same reasons, a physician will not define his or her capacity as "a counselor to the dying," in the manner of Kübler-Ross, because if the patient is not a candidate for aggressive treatment (and hence outside the population of the dying), neither is he or she a candidate for verbal exploration of the fears of the dying. Even the physician who says, "It is our job to help a patient to die," means something different from the confrontation of euthanasia. He or she means, "We are running out of options to offer this patient. How are we to care for the patient without destroying the hope that there is still one powerful option to offer?" Talk of options is talk of living.

As has been suggested, the subtle social dimensions of the decision whether or not to treat aggressively are buried in the clinical data. The law of the stranger has already been introduced. The patient about whom you know nothing but who has an immediate need for aggressive measures (resuscitation, a pacing wire, emergency surgery) is treated to the fullest possible extent. Once additional information is acquired (the patient has baseline dementia; the patient is a chronic alcoholic with lung cancer; the patient has disseminated cancer), limitations are established: "We shall do up to x, but then no more." This means that the staff will plow on, waiting for total system failure, in conditions of incomplete information or where secondary medical problems are irrelevant to viability. Such patients are deemed "salvageable." Where further information detracts from the patient's assumed "salvageability," the patient becomes "nonsalvageable," and support rather than treatment becomes the rule.

The second constraint on medical "heroics" is the presence or absence of a visible family network. It can document the patient's social viability and influence physicians who waver in their aggressiveness. It can also contribute to the decision to minimize aggressiveness, if the patient impresses upon the house staff his wish for minimal support. The absence of a visible family can invoke the law of the stranger, to the extent that medical resources are in abundance, or it can mean that the patient without a family loses the respirator to another patient who has visitors constantly in attendance beseeching the physician to "do something."

> An elderly Italian patriarch lay dying with his daughters and sons in constant attendance. The MICU staff spoke of "the vigil." His family was able to convince the staff to remove the tubes and IV lines which were the means to a prolonged dying, even

though the staff thought it conceivable that he might return home, though bedridden with little chance of ever getting up.

Louise Marks benefited from a visible family network. Her son was in continual communication with her physicians; he was a frequent visitor to his mother's bedside. He repeatedly communicated his wish that his mother be kept comfortable but that no unusual procedures be tried.

When there appears to be no effective constraint on "heroics," the situation can become ludicrous, as was the case with a fifty-year-old black woman who had been having brain seizures for forty-eight hours, and who had a fever in the range of 104°F, along with kidney failure and an unidentified micro-organism in her blood and urine cultures. Everyone was writing consultation notes about her "grim prognosis." George Smith, the fourth-year student, went so far as to admit that the signs of her having significant brain stem function were decreasing each day. He recounted his resident's comment of the previous night: "This lady's mission in life is to be teaching material for interns. As long as she lives, we do everything we can." When I asked Brian Marshall, the resident, why they were working so hard on Elsie Carter, he replied, "Elsie is reversible if we can stop her seizures and get her kidneys working." For two more days Elsie Carter required intensive nursing and the better part of George Smith's time and attention.

Both Louise Marks and Elsie Carter died in a university teaching hospital in a big city, where a wealth of technology was available to maintain a patient as long as the physicians wished to employ it or until it no longer made any difference. The cases were unexceptional with regard to diagnosis and management. More important, they illustrate the medical perspective on death. For the physician in this context death is not an event; it is a process that is common to all illness. Within fiction and within our personal experiences, death is an abrupt event, a termination of a life. But within the hospital it is everywhere and nowhere, for the wise physician knows that he or she cannot predict death, only the momentum toward death. Some deaths are more welcome than others.

At times the layperson assumes that the physician can control and predict death; but physicians are sometimes wrong in their management and inaccurate in their predictions, so there is no assurance of when and how death will occur. Yet by comparison with the incapacity of the layperson to hold back death, the physician appears both powerful and knowing. Perhaps if we expected less omnipotence and omniscience from our physicians, we would be less disappointed in their humanity. Furthermore, when a patient asks his physician, "Am I going to die?" and the doctor says, "No, I am going to make you better," the patient assumes he is lying; it is only a matter of when he shall die and then he will prove the physician wrong. The physician, on the other hand, knows that the patient will die, but he does not know when. So he assumes it is no lie to answer no. The physician knows that if he does not claim to be improving the patient's condition, the patient will worry that he really is dying. So both patient and physician get trapped in their expectations of each other.

The technological face of death has created problems where none previously existed. In this regard, these two deaths were exemplary, for without technology neither Louise Marks nor Elsie Carter would have lain in her bed waiting for death with the hum of machinery in her ears. Consider the enormity of the change that has occurred since respirators and cardiac pacemakers became part of the armamentarium against death.

When people died at home without the benefit of respirators and dialysis, without oxygen tanks and inhalation therapy, without cobalt treatments and arterial catheterizations, there was no question of needlessly and painfully prolonging life. When the body could no longer function on its own, it "gave up the ghost." Notions of "a good death" were tied to social life and oftentimes were bounded by one's fears for one's soul and the need to find spiritual repair before the inevitable disrepair of the body.[16] The idea of "death with dignity"[17] could only mean using one's dying to teach one's successors that there was nothing to fear in death. With the decline of religious belief in the everlasting life of the soul or some form of bodily resurrection, death ceased to be a means to an end (eternal life or damnation), and became an end in itself. Furthermore, when death moved from the bedroom to the hospital ward, it ceased to be a private, personal matter and became subject to the contrivances of bureaucratic organization. And with the manifest benefits of medical technology came certain disadvantages: death was no longer wholly in the hands of God or nature, but subject to the ability of men and women to intervene and prevent its finality.

Where there is the ability to stave off death, there is power;

moreover, power is further increased when death ceases to be a way-station to some higher goal. Power has meaning when it is tested and triumphs over weakness; where it exists as potentiality it is illusive. It is commonly held that power should not extend beyond the range necessary to accomplish its goal. To use a machine gun to kill a deer is an abuse of power, when a single shot would do as well. Some would argue that hunting deer is an abuse of power, except to prevent starvation.

To use the total armamentarium of modern medicine to keep a comatose, terminally ill patient alive may be interpreted as a similar abuse of power, particularly the more apparent it becomes that nothing will have any real effect on the extent or quality of life available to the dying person. If the quality of survival is enhanced, then one may be more cautious in claiming abuse. But in this context death is no longer a matter between a human being and the totality of body systems, between a person and his or her God. It becomes a public document of the concluding battle between persons judged qualified to redress the deterioration of the body and those who look on without the capacity to do anything more than cry "enough." Consequently, those in the latter position will frequently feel that too much or not enough has been done for their loved ones. They will continually seek some rule that will move the decisions out of the hands of the powerful into the hands of the less powerful; for then they, too, will have done something for the dying. And, perhaps, once the rule is securely upheld, they will not have to witness this painful scene again and again with the loss of each family member. So one tactic is to seek to overturn the standards of action that serve the physician, who seems to have power over life and death, by resorting to the courts. They invoke the language of rights and address the courts to recognize a right to die. The substitution of moral rhetoric for an analysis of issues as they occur in their natural context is an attempt to find a meaningful way of dealing with an apparently insolvable problem, the appropriation of power by physicians.

The "right to die" is actually a "right to *let* die," for it has meaning only in the context of imminent demise. The Karen Quinlan case (137 N.J. Superior Court, 227) is the embodiment of this principle. At University Hospital the case of Zhudi Dov, a charming, gracious man of eighty-two who liked to quote Keats and Shelley, was an additional example of this problem. He was convinced he was dying,

TABLE 3

Case of Louise Marks:
"Right to Die" of Comatose Sixty-eight-year-old Female

Clinical
Issues

(1) clinical prognosis of patient*
    (a) probability of organ function*
    (b) probability of mental function*
    (c) probability of social function
(2) Cardiac status after removal of pacing wire*

Legal
Issues

(1) Existence of "right to die"
(2) With whom does the determination of extensiveness of medical support rest?†
    (a) patient
    (b) family†
    (c) representative of religious organization, e.g., priest
    (d) physicians†
    (e) some combination of the above†
(3) Existence of "right to refuse treatment"†
(4) Existence of "right to privacy"
(5) Existence of "right of self-determination"
(6) Contributory negligence of physician
(7) Legal precedent for euthanasia

Ethical
Issues

(1) Right to sustain life for life's sake†
    (a) wishes of patient prior to illness*
    (b) wishes of family*
    (c) wishes of physicians
    (d) societal interest in sustaining life
(2) Scarce and limited medical resources—their allocation
(3) Who shall decide who lives?
(4) Under what conditions should medical support be withdrawn from a comatose patient?
    (a) clinical criteria†
    (b) mental criteria†
    (c) social criteria†
(5) How can one determine the needs of a dying person?
    (a) psychological needs
    (b) social needs†
    (c) biological needs†

* Addressed by physicians through stated perspective.
† Addressed by physicians, but not through stated perspective.

despite the insistence of the staff that he would live for several more years. But he had ceased to rage against the misfortunes of life and looked forward to death. He successfully refused to undergo heart surgery because he felt he had lived long enough. He was not yet in the condition of Louise Marks, but the succeeding months would bring him closer.

Table 3 illustrates the clinical, legal, and ethical issues in the Marks case. The expression of the perspectives is clinical, moral, and legal, though significantly more weight is given to the clinical perspective than to either the moral or the legal perspective.

The first two cases illustrated the issues of informed consent and the constraint of individual autonomy resulting from the medical assignation of mental impairment, either through emotional disturbance or genetic mutation. In the first instance, the ethical issues were blatantly ignored; in the second, they were ineffectually addressed. In both cases there was informal acknowledgment that legal issues imposed limitations on professional behavior, but the extent of those limitations was manipulated by going through the motions of fulfilling the legal stipulations. Sadie Myers gave her informed consent; her signature is on the appropriate piece of paper. The parents of Joan Spoon gave their consent to her cardiac catheterization and as her guardians would probably have faced no difficulty in obtaining her sterilization. (Her case was referred to the Patients' Rights Committee, though further information was not made available to me.) In the clinical setting, both cases are unspectacular, representing myriad cases with ethical components of consent, responsibility, autonomy, and values.

The case of Louise Marks advanced some of the same issues as the first two, but in the context of the terminally ill patient. It also introduced a new factor, social death, as an infringement on human autonomy. Social death occurs when the patient is treated *as if* she or he had already died. Such patients are frequently referred to in the past tense by relatives at the bedside: ''He was a good man, you know?'' A patient who is the object of social death has the capacity neither for informed consent nor for discussion of personal autonomy, which creates a situation where the decisions of what to do fall to the senior ranking house officer, after consultation with the attending physician and private physician (if there is one).

4 Charting Ethics

These three cases have been used to demonstrate the existence of ethical issues in clinical practice. They have as their common denominator the issue of informed consent. In addition, they demonstrate the manner in which medical designations, such as endogeneous depression, effectively constrain patient autonomy as a condition of the patient-physician relationship. This constraint goes beyond the classical obligations of the sick role, as described by Talcott Parsons.[1] Rather, it suggests that medicalization of a complaint confers on the physician enormous power, which exercised to the fullest consists of the substitution of physician autonomy for patient autonomy. When the physician decides for the patient what should be done for him or her, based on the tacit consent of the patient or the patient's representatives, the physician usurps the prerogatives of the patient to question or to seek additional opinions. This usurpation is made easier by the patient's passivity.

Another way of looking at this relationship is to acknowledge that people with medical profiles similar to those of the three women, who do not avail themselves of medical assistance, maintain their autonomy. Undoubtedly people in this category may be limited in their capacity to exercise autonomy by virtue of mental or physical deficiencies, but their limitations do not negate their autonomy. Psychiatrists refer to "the walking wounded," or to those people with emotional impairments who cope without benefit of psychiatric services. There are women who are mentally deficient by virtue of I.Q., with and without Down's Syndrome as the source of that deficiency, who retain their capacity to reproduce. Finally, people do die without physicians mediating between them and death, though the association of hospitals and death is commonplace.

The relationship between femaleness and autonomy is another theme from these three cases. My selection of three female patients as principal examples was accidental, though it is common knowledge that women seek medical care more frequently than men.[2] The most common explanations include the following: women have more time than men to visit doctors because they are unemployed or employed only part time; women as mothers see physicians more frequently than men because of their children's illnesses, and this makes them more familiar with the medical system, which encourages their use of it; women have too much leisure time to indulge in psychoneurotic complaints which cause them to seek medical care.

While Otto Pollak calls the following explanation "a twentieth-century theory of hysteria,"[3] it is one way of looking at the problems which affect women as health-care consumers. In addition, it illuminates the problems of men. Female patients may be victims of a double bind, the receivers of contradictory expectations on the part of society, and of physicians in particular. Women have been taught that aggressive behavior is "unfeminine," but they are routinely chastised by husbands and other family members for doing nothing about their physical complaints, once recommendations to end their complaining prove ineffective. They therefore attempt to do something about their problems by seeking medical attention, an act of "unnatural aggressiveness." They are then cast in a dependent role by physicians and are castigated for wasting the physician's time with their minor complaints. They are sent home with the advice not to worry and told to return if their condition worsens. Meanwhile, the latent reasons why muscular-skeletal aches or nervousness should loom so large in these women's lives is ignored as outside the relevant skills of the physician in the university hospital setting. Women's attempts at autonomy are treated as a source of professional annoyance. Women are confounded by the contradictory messages to "do something" and to "do nothing" as a condition of their acceptability as women. The role contradictions that women experience when they seek medical counsel for the aches and pains of social discomfort may also explain why men are slow to seek medical aid for such problems as drug abuse and hypertension. Intrinsically they sense that the patient "role" will create contradictions with masculinity which cannot be resolved without changing physician behavior or notions of "masculinity."

The three cases also demonstrate the distinction between *pro-*

fessional ethics, as used by physicians, and *ethical issues,* as used by the laity. The first consists of standards of performance maintained by physicians through the use of rewards and sanctions as a means of social control within professional circles. These are fairly broad principles of acceptable behavior, exemplified in the American Medical Association's Code.[4] A corollary to the most general formulation of professional standards of behavior is the protection of self-interest. The physician may bend or break the rules as long as he or she ensures the low visibility of the offense by protecting superiors and patients from knowledge of purposeful deviance.

Ethical issues, as used by nonphysicians, consist of situations that evoke the need for ethical discussion based on a personal system of morals. While the two need not be in conflict, the physician tends to be blind to the ethical issues as long as the plan of management can be reduced to concrete data, derived from a professional orientation toward pathology and organicity. The physician may decide that the patient with no cardiac or renal function, who is dependent on a respirator for each breath, is going to die regardless of anything that can be done; and so the physician turns his or her attention to patients who have less chance of dying during the house officer's rotation. The layperson may also agree that "the patient should be allowed to die" without knowing the organic basis for the physician's pessimism. What becomes newsworthy, however, is the case in which physicians and laypersons disagree on the probability of the patient's demise, with laypersons arguing for the termination of efforts, while physicians favor aggressive action. Once again, the physician cites the status of body systems and relevant literature to argue in favor of clinical activity; the layperson cites "the immorality of suffering" and urges the cessation of medical heroics.

Another theme common to these three cases needs to be spelled out as a means of underscoring the arbitrariness evidenced in the narratives. Even when patients have private physicians, their primary physicians are house officers and medical students assigned to their service. To some extent the cast of characters determines the course of events. This is true of clinical preferences as well as concern (or lack of concern) with ethical issues. While generalizations have been offered pertaining to how many students or house officers tend to act in a given situation, they are not ironclad rules of action.

The nurses in the Medical Intensive Care Unit repeatedly referred to the resident who had preceded Fatolah Paz, seven weeks prior to my arrival. Harold Rosner believed so strongly in aggressive medicine that only death could convince him to stop. The story was told of how Harold arrived in the MICU and found Jerry Jones comatose. He gave Jerry Jones mouth-to-mouth resuscitation and revived him. He then learned that Jerry had "the red snapper" or active tuberculosis in addition to his other medical problems. Nevertheless, during the month-long rotation, Harold resuscitated Jerry Jones eight times, which was something of a record by the nurses' accounts. He finally died during the eighth emergency code call. They reported that they were relieved when Harold left the service because they frequently believed that his aggressiveness violated good sense. They had more confidence in his successor's judgment, though they did not necessarily agree with everything he did. The resident who ran the MICU during the last three weeks of my presence evoked these stories from the nurses when he persisted in treating Elsie Carter aggressively, despite her repeated seizures and total kidney failure.

Part of the ambiguity the physician feels arises from the historical events which have transformed medical practice. The number of options available to a physician today are many times the number available to the physician of twenty years ago. Dialysis, for example, has advanced from an exorbitantly expensive and experimental procedure to an established part of medical practice. Furthermore, the availability of kidney dialysis machines is no longer limited to university medical centers. Home dialysis and local dialysis centers offer a specialized function of chronic dialysis. Aside from dialysis, there is the possibility of organ transplantation. The technology of kidney transplants is so advanced that the greatest obstacle is the unavailability of usable organs. Finally, patients are aware of the possibility of kidney transplants, so they may exert influence on physicians who in other circumstances would not entertain the possibility. For example, the rural physician may not have admission privileges at a hospital equipped to do kidney transplants, but with advances in communication and transportation he or she may be able to offer the patient this option with the cooperation of a regional facility. Decisions, even purely clinical ones, were simpler in a pretechnological era. Even as early as the discovery of sulfa drugs, a burgeoning number of choices began to confront the physician with a patient in renal failure.

Ethical issues in the clinical setting vary from the unobserved,

to those transformed into medical-legal questions, to those acknowledged on their own terms. There are many gradations in-between,
suggesting a continuum of visibility. Furthermore, the visibility-in-
visibility of ethical issues may vary with individual physicians. It may
also vary with individual services which take their tone from the
influential men and women who can encourage or discourage concern
with ethical issues. There is evidence to suggest that some subpopulations
of physicians, such as newly appointed house officers, may have more
difficulty discerning the relevance of a moral perspective than other
groups of physicians, such as attending physicians. Additional research
might substantiate a hypothesis that medical specialists vary with respect
to their concern with ethical issues in medicine, with those who have
substantial numbers of chronically ill patients more likely to invoke the
moral perspective than their colleagues who deal with acutely ill patients.

Medical students who observe how attending physicians and
house officers act in situations like the ones enumerated here acquire a
similar demeanor or suffer much discomfort. Since students' role models are often unaware of the ethical issues or confused about how to
handle them, students cannot resolve their own confusion by looking
to their elders. Consequently, students learn to use the clinical perspective as their dominant perspective. The modifications that occur, requiring the use of the legal and moral perspectives, seem to appear in
the later phases of their socialization. The next three chapters will
elaborate further the clinical, legal, and ethical perspectives.

PART TWO

Three Perspectives

5 The Clinical Perspective

In our culture, in contrast to simpler ones, when a layperson comes up against a problem that cannot be resolved by common sense (which itself is based on prior experience), he or she turns to experts. The supposition is made that experts have the answers, which they calculate according to fixed rules of problem-solving. Quite frequently one assumes that expertise is based on special education as well as experience, so one expects the expert to bring a set of complex formulations to bear on the problem, which the layperson does not expect to understand except in simplified form. When a pipe springs a leak, most people call a plumber to repair it. They do not expect the plumber to tell them why he does what he does, and they do not question how he goes about his work. They are satisfied if the pipe is returned to working condition.

It is becoming increasingly common, however, for laypersons to question the actions of physicians. One wants to know the whys and hows of surgery before giving consent, while in previous decades one was more likely to accept the physician's recommendation on the grounds that physicians, by virtue of their degree, know what they are doing. Laypersons, however, have become much more sophisticated about medicine through the media, and this gives them a basis for challenging physicians. Today when parents challenge the physician's assumption of their child's need for a tonsillectomy, they use their own judgment to question the physician's clinical judgment. The parents' judgment may be called *nonclinical judgment,* which is the rank ordering of values based on individual experience and psychological inclination devoid of any professional bias. *Clinical judgment* is the capacity to make medical decisions based on clinical data (history, physical examination, diagnosis, and prognosis), with support from secondary resources, such as the medical literature.

We may expand this ideal of personal, or nonclinical, judgment into the concept of a moral perspective, for the parent is actually asking, What is the right thing to do? The parent formulates two parts to the question: What is the right thing for me to do as a parent— consent or refuse consent for a tonsillectomy for my child? What is the right thing for the physician to do—recommend surgery or another course of treatment? Without professional expertise to evaluate the competence of the physician, except for some superficial knowledge based on newsweeklies and other media sources, the parent must evaluate the patient-physician relationship on nonprofessional terms. Therefore, the parent accepts or rejects the physician's clinical judgment on grounds determined by interpersonal satisfaction: (1) manifestations by the physician of interest in the child's problems; (2) recommendations by friends, the family physician, or other family members in support of the physician's competence; (3) expressions of satisfaction by other patients in the waiting room with the physician's past performance; and a (4) temperamental match between parent and physician. While none of the factors alone seems to be sufficient reason for agreeing with the physician's recommendation for surgery, taken together they seem to have considerable weight. The conflict between the personal, scientifically uninformed perspective of the parent and the clinical perspective of the physician can be resolved by sufficient social grounds in support of the fiduciary relationship.

When we look at how physicians solve problems in the medical setting, we find that they invoke a particular mode of thinking and argument that is universally shared by university-trained physicians. In the next several chapters we will have many opportunities to see examples of the clinical perspective and the process by which it is acquired. As subsequent anecdotes will show, physicians find it irrelevant to use terms like *right* and *wrong*. Rather than ask whether it is "right" to give a diabetic patient insulin, they would want to establish whether the *extent of the patient's problem* (insufficient production of insulin by the pancreas) *necessitates* daily injections of insulin or whether management by dietary restriction would suffice. The question for them would be, What is the appropriate treatment? which in medical jargon is known as "the treatment of choice." While they might find themselves in extensive debate over the identification of the treatment of choice, they would resolve the issue by appealing to concrete, highly circumscribed evidence rather than to moral judgments, although in some instances perspectives can be seen to overlap or blur.

So far I have argued that there is a discrepancy in education and experience between patient and physician which prevents them from solving problems in similar ways. The fundamental inequality of patient and physician is expressed in situations where the patient disagrees with the physician's recommendation. The patient enunciates his or her personal judgment in moral terms, while the physician invokes the clinical perspective. While the physician may seek to persuade the patient by elaborating and simplifying the clinical reasons for his recommendation, the issue is likely to be resolved ultimately by the presence or absence of social reasons validating the competence of the physician. If the patient can find reason from friends, family, or a trusted medical advisor to believe that "Charles Allen, M.D., is a top-notch physician to whom I would send a member of my own family," the patient's arguments and resistance will dissipate in most cases.

We will also want to look at situations where the physician cannot resolve a problem by appeal to clinical knowledge, chiefly because the clinical options have been exhausted. For example, what can a physician do for a patient dying from cancer once the disease has infiltrated more than one organ system? If the patient's suffering is prolonged, the physician must consider what can be done to alleviate the pain. The most common situation is the need to weigh the risk of depressing respiratory function by high dosages of morphine, or restricting the patient to "safe" dosages without fully relieving the pain. The physician must consider his legal responsibilities to the patient, lest he or she be guilty of killing the patient through an excessive dose of narcotics. With the exhaustion of the clinical perspective, the physician may need to consider the legal perspective. And if the physician should decide either that there is no basis for fear of a lawsuit or that there are grounds to fear prosecution but the slim probability of conviction is worth risking, he or she may then justify the actions taken in terms of the moral perspective. The alleviation of suffering at the risk of mortality in a person racked by cancer then assumes a higher order of obligation than the need to limit medication to nonaddictive and nonthreatening levels of effectiveness.

There can be agreement among the perspectives, as well as conflict; until recently we expected consensus. However, situations of conflict are becoming increasingly common because expanding medical technology creates problems where none previously existed. Where previously physicians could cure patients or preserve them in the same state, they now can also preserve them in drastically altered states. This gives rise to a troublesome and confusing situation. Now that physicians can sustain "human vegetables" long after social function has ceased, they are caught in a problem of cultural lag. They have neither the clinical expertise to revitalize patients nor sufficient experience in dealing with situations that are without clearly articulated rules of performance. At times medical progress outstrips the pace of change in social norms, so that physicians face dilemmas that are not governed by generalized social sanctions, which might make the proposed action more discernibly "right" or "wrong." Often the question of what to do is resolved by doing nothing, which alleviates physician discomfort with uncertainty, by allowing nature to take its course.

While waiting to decide whether to submit a patient to emergency surgery, the house staff find that the patient has "slipped away," sparing them the need to evaluate whether extensive senility diminishes the benefits of surgery. By delaying phototherapy, with its unknown long-term effects, physicians can wait and see whether the condition of the jaundiced infant improves dramatically and thus negates the need for "bili-lights," or worsens and forces their hand.* In either case, waiting enables the physician to let the situation reveal a course of action, while minimizing the need to raise questions with ethical or legal overtones that are not clearly answered in the clinical literature.

In situations like these, medical students may recognize the conflicting role demands without perceiving any satisfactory way of resolving them. Their role models also lack clear solutions to the complex questions facing them. While the students' medical education

*In phototherapy, the baby is put into an isolette outfitted with special lights called "bili-lights." Such therapy reduces the bilirubin level, which is determined by a simple blood test. While the biochemical explanation for why phototherapy seems to reduce the bilirubin level, and thus alleviate the threat of brain damage, is undeveloped, the practice has gained widespread acceptance in university teaching hospitals.

may be directed toward adopting the clinical perspective as *the* problem-solving perspective, there may be sufficient numbers of unsettling experiences to suggest the poverty of clinical thinking in providing satisfactory ways of coping with problematic situations. During their clinical rotations students see that physicians adopt various ways of coping with the limitations of the clinical perspective, such as joking, set-speeches, and avoidance. But there is little direct confrontation with the sources of discomfort.

In forthcoming chapters the problem-solving techniques of physicians will be contrasted with those of laypersons in a clinical situation. Since laypersons are more apt to apply a moral perspective than either a legal or a clinical one, they lack the means to negotiate with physicians when conflict becomes apparent. Also, because they invoke a single perspective instead of two or three, they tend to see the question in terms of right and wrong, which reduces the muddled quality of the actual dilemma. Furthermore, we shall note that competition among perspectives does not imply the superiority of one perspective over another. Sometimes it does not entail the complete ascendancy of one perspective over another, such as when the moral and legal issues become blurred. Nevertheless, we shall have to consider which perspective is used by whom, and under what conditions. Ultimately we shall see that the clinical perspective is used most frequently; the internalization of this clinical perspective is of critical importance in the training of physicians.

Contemporary concern with medical practice and the use of the clinical perspective by physicians is derived from vast changes in the technological level of medicine. Laypersons tend to perceive moral questions in clinical situations, where physicians see only clinical problems. But this one facet of historical change is symbolic of more pervasive changes in professional knowledge. For not only does medicine change, but so do law and morals. We are inclined to think of "the law," or "medicine," or "morals" as fixed entities. In reality each is subject to social change, which makes them dynamic concepts. The interlocking nature of these changes is demonstrated by the issue of abortion, as well as other issues impinging on reproductive capacity (artificial insemination by donor, sterilization, and contraception). Changes in medical technology, such as the technique of saline abortion and vacuum extraction of the fetus, have effected changes in the law, which has made abortions legal and available to many women who formerly were unable to obtain them. But regardless of the existing technology, without moral tolerance, abortions would not have become the subject of a Supreme Court ruling. While the performance of abortions has been part of history, public acceptance of them and of women who have them is a recent phenomenon within American society. Without changes in public morality, new technology could not come to light; and without the two, there would be no need to modify the law.

We can treat each of the three perspectives (the clinical, the legal, and the moral) as a range, with the clinical range as the first to be discussed. It is a way of expressing the underlying social change affecting the practice of medicine in University Hospital. Subsequently, we shall look at the legal perspective, and then the moral perspective. These ranges may be treated as ideal types, with the poles as conceptual ideals; that is, there are no pure cases in existence which embody the described polarities. Instead, there is increasing predominance of one ideal type over another as one moves to either extreme on the range.

For purposes of discussion we can describe a range of clinical practice, with poles of experimentation (clinical investigation) and of common practice:

Clinical Investigation ⟵⟶ Common Practice

If we wish to be more inclusive in a description of clinical practice, we might extend the range past common practice to an ultimate pole of obsolescence, where a procedure which at some time in the past was experimental has now ceased to be part of common practice and may in fact be discouraged as "bad" practice.

Clinical Investigation ⟵⟶ Common Practice (⟶ Obsolescence)

While we readily speak of the gradual adoption of a given technique or practice by physicians as it moves out of experimentation, we tend to forget many medical procedures which have ceased to be common medical practice, and which have dropped from collective memory as ever having been the treatment of choice. For example, during the late nineteenth century female circumcision was used as a means of behavior control and as the treatment of choice for many mental and physical problems common to women during that period.[1] Medical practice is treated as a range, because no single medical therapy is wholly experimental or universally common practice. It is obvious that experimental modalities of therapy are predicated on practices which are part of the medical canon. Swine flu vaccine grew out of existing knowledge of innoculations, dating from Jenner. The obverse is true as well. The most common of practices, the administration of aspirin for headaches, contains an element of the experimental, for while it may alleviate the pain it may also induce gastric upset. The repeated success of aspirin in curing headaches will lead the patient to conclude that aspirin is an effective remedy for headache pain.

This range of medical practice, with its poles of experimentation and common practice, is used by Renée Fox and Judith Swazey in *The Courage to Fail,* an examination of organ transplants and dialysis. Furthermore, with a discussion of the clinical moratorium on heart transplantation, they document the uneven temperament of this process of introduction and adaptation. At times it seems to proceed by quantum jumps.[2] The course of kidney dialysis demonstrates this. The first kidney machine was built in the early 1940s by Dr. Willem Kolff. By 1950 at least three American hospitals had artificial kidney machines. In 1960 the longest reported survival of a patient on a hemodialysis machine was 181 days. But with the use of a semipermanent connecting tube called the Scribner shunt, the possibility of long-term dialysis was enhanced. A further advance in 1966, the fistula system (sewing an artery to a vein), created a permanent site for needles without requiring an exposed shunt. The survival period has been extended to more than eight years.[3]

Less commonly considered is the process by which a procedure falls from favor. For example, while a majority of house officers on the medical services of University Hospital still subscribe to the use of "blow bottles" as part of therapy for pneumonia or chronic obstructed pulmonary disease, Dr. Murphy, the attending physician for the pulmonary consultation service, grew angry whenever he saw the plastic bottles by the bedside. The object is for the patient to blow a blue fluid out of one bottle and into the other by forcing air into the connecting tubing, which acts as a siphon. This forces the patient to take deep breaths in order to break up congestion in the lungs. Dr. Murphy argued that this is ineffectual and deceivingly simple-minded therapy, because for the better part of the day the patient continues to breathe incorrectly. He preferred that his students stand by the patient and coach him or her in taking deep breaths and to urge the patient to integrate this behavior into his or her convalescence. Undoubtedly, students who train under him will influence others that blow bottles no longer have a place in respiratory therapy. Thus, procedures that were once the treatment of choice slip into acceptable practice before becoming minority practice as they make their way toward obsolescence.

The university house officer's lack of regard for the local physician, the LMD, is in part derived from the LMD's slowness to adopt innovative practices or even his lack of knowledge of what is the treatment of choice within university circles. In terms of the house officer's perspective, which readily becomes the student's perspective, it appears that patients get inferior care in the hands of the LMD, compared to what they might receive in the university setting.

This is not to say that all LMDs are regarded as incompetent. On occasion a local physician will be commended for thoroughness or astuteness of diagnosis, though the tenor of the remarks will contain an element of surprise at such a performance. Academic medicine is characterized by compulsive thoroughness that is both time-consuming and expensive—and consequently not part of the LMD's standard of care as a routine matter. This compulsive thoroughness may justify academic medicine through its support of an ethic of comprehensive medical care.

The treatment of choice is the therapy that is offered to the patient as the common practice by the community of physicians who engage in this sector of medical practice. For instance, when the bilirubin level climbs, the neonatologist considers the use of bililights. However, depending on place of training he or she may consider a specific level as requiring or failing to require putting the baby under the lights.[4] While neonatologists may vary in their determination of the danger threshold, they will concur on the appropriateness of the treatment once that threshold is crossed.

This kind of situation divides physicians into two sorts. The first, when faced with a difficult situation, prefers to do something and is likely to have an earlier threshold of action. Such physicians prefer to do something even if the task has no intrinsic medical meaning, like running down to a lab to see whether test results are in, rather than wait out the crisis. The second sort of physician, faced with the same situation, prefers to do nothing, hoping that in time a clear course of action will become apparent.

When a patient is jointly managed by surgeons and "medicine

men," there is often underlying conflict over the treatment of choice, based on their professional biases. The surgeon prefers to cure surgically rather than to wait and treat pharmacologically, because surgery gives results that are immediate and clear. The bias of the person trained in medicine is to exhaust pharmacological management before resorting to surgery, because it does not have the risks of anesthesia and surgical morbidity. Also, surgery is frequently irreversible, and "medicine men" may be more inclined to maintain the integrity of the body than surgeons, who by definition violate its integrity.

For example, a patient on the medical service was suffering from postsurgical complications which required medical management of his electrolyte balance and his fluid retention levels. Instead of getting better, his condition worsened, and the house staff debated whether "a tap," a surgical incision into the chest cavity, might provide information on the probable source and identity of his infection as well as allow them to drain some of the excess fluid his body was retaining.

Attending physician: What are the risks in this guy?

Resident: People die.

Attending physician: What do they die from?

Intern: People die from cutting an artery while doing the tap.

Attending physician: We can continue to treat the problem medically. But we need to know whether we are going to benefit from knowing what kind of fluid he has in his chest . . . in terms of surgical therapy, we might want to know. You can control his infection, but only if you know what it is through doing a tap.

Diagnostically, it was argued, a tap would provide the reason for any subsequent deterioration in his condition. If they continued to treat him medically, they would lose information that would be very valuable if he decompensated, or continually failed to regulate the fluid load in his body, so that his heart, lungs, and kidneys would have to work too hard. If he did decompensate, it would be too late to wonder about the nature of his infection. The debate was never resolved, and the resident passed around photocopies of five articles on the management of this condition. Later in the day, the decision was reached by the attending physician to send the patient to surgery. The patient died in surgery.

The range of clinical practice demonstrates the complexity of clinical decision-making. The "premie" (premature infant) intensive care unit offered a relevant case of experimentation.

Baby Girl Brown was born weighing 780 grams* and with a gestational age of 24–26 weeks. At one minute she had been given an Apgar of 1, at five minutes, 4.† It had been a breech presentation.‡ Physically the baby was quite immature in appearance and in the tenth decile for its size and weight.

On talking with the obstetricians who had delivered the Brown baby, the premie team learned that they had considered it a hopeless case. The chief had exercised his prerogative not to administer steroids to the mother in an attempt to stop her labor and to allow the fetus a few more weeks of maturation. Baby Girl Brown had the distinction of being the smallest baby brought into the premie intensive care nursery in the memory of the staff.

It was expected that if the baby survived into the fifth or sixth hour, she would suffer from Respiratory Distress Syndrome (RDS), an impairment of respiratory function due to the rudimentary development of the newborn's lungs, in particular, the air sacs or alveoli. One hour after birth, the resident decided to put in an umbilical line, an intravenous line through the umbilicus, and to order blood for an exchange transfusion. In an exchange transfusion, fresh whole blood is slowly given to the infant, while equal quantities of her blood are slowly removed. There is always the danger of overloading the infant's circulatory system with too high a volume of fluids, and thus throwing the intricate balance of electrolytes out of kilter as well as making the kidneys, lungs, and heart work too hard to reestablish equilibrium. Baby Girl Brown was to come under the research protocol of Dr. Maria Ramos, head of neonatology. She had established criteria for

---

*780 grams is approximately 1 pound, 11.5 ounces. A baby must weigh 2040 grams (4 lb., 8 oz.) before it can be discharged to go home.

†The Apgar score is the evaluation of the newborn infant's physical status by assigning numerical values to heart rate, respiratory effort, muscle tone, reflex irritability, and skin color. Scores of 10, 9, and 8 simply require conservation of body heat; scores of 5, 6, and 7 generally mean that if the infant is suctioned, warmed, and given some oxygen, survival is likely; scores of less than 5 express the probability of infant mortality despite assistance.

‡A breech presentation occurs if any part of the pelvic extremity of the fetus or the buttocks is presented, rather than the head or other part of the upper body.

the selection of RDS babies for exchange transfusions in which a donor's blood, probably the father's, which is less than twenty-four hours old, and optimally less than eight hours old, is given to the newborn in order to enhance his or her chances of adequate respiratory function.

When Mrs. Brown came into the nursery, Bill Lash, the intern, sat down with her and talked with her about her daughter's condition. He explained how serious it was and what was being done for her. He told the mother that they wanted to give the baby an exchange transfusion, that it was an experimental procedure, and that babies who received this treatment seemed to have better chances for survival than those who did not. The mother did not actually read the standard forms (forms 4 and 5), for her mind was already set on doing whatever Bill Lash said had to be done to keep her baby alive. She gave her "optimistic consent."

All the time the baby was in an incubator breathing a combination of oxygen and nitrogen, she was benefiting from what had once been experimental and then innovative procedure. Modifications had occurred in the proportion of oxygen employed, for in the late 1940s and early 1950s it had been discovered that too high an oxygen concentration caused retrolental fibroplasia, a deterioration of the retina that sometimes caused blindness. It is now the treatment of choice to put premature babies who have immature lungs into this artificial environment in order to allow them the necessary time to mature and acquire healthy alveolar functioning.

By Dr. Ramos's observation, 90 percent treated with exchange transfusions survived; this was exceedingly high and the best rate in the country. For the next three days the team hovered between amazement that the tiny infant continued to survive and grim pessimism as she failed to thrive. She suffered from increasingly lengthy periods of apnea, or spells when respiration stopped. She died on the third day, after another exchange transfusion.

Rounds with Dr. Ramos were in turn dramatic, Socratic, and dogmatic. She stressed that "these are thinking rounds and not factual rounds." She demanded that her students confront the realities of medicine, including an awareness of the degree of unknown risk inherent in common procedures: "Listen how this backfires on you if you haven't been thinking about every move. . . . You must think through the pros and cons of acts which are taken as naive solutions." At one

FORM 4

THE CHILDREN'S HOSPITAL
GENERAL CONSENT FORM

Authority for Diagnosis, Treatment, and Transportation

I hereby grant permission for such diagnostic procedures and treatment as may be deemed necessary or advisable by the physician in charge of the patient.

I consent to the transportation of the patient between University Hospital and The Children's Hospital. Any and all such transportation may be made whenever deemed necessary or advisable by the physician in charge of the patient.

I hereby certify that I am related to said patient as follows:. . . . .
    Witness   Signed . . . .

. . . .   Address: . . . .

I authorize The Children's Hospital to release the patient in the custody of my spouse upon discharge
    Witness   Signed . . . .

. . . .   Address: . . . .

Authority for Operation

I hereby grant permission to Dr. . . . ., his assistants or designees to perform such operative procedures as are, in his or their professional judgment, desirable to relieve the conditions described above and any other conditions from which the patient may be suffering, whether or not now known.

I consent to the administration of anesthesia and to the use of such anesthetics as may be deemed advisable in connection with such procedures. I consent to performance of an exchange or replacement blood transfusion when the patient's condition requires it. I consent to the performance of cardiac catheterizations or other special diagnostic procedures required.

These operative procedures may be performed in The Children's Hospital, The University Hospital, or the Community Hospital of the University, at the discretion of the attending physicians.

I hereby certify that I am related to said patient as follows:. . . . .

    Witness   Signed: . . . .

. . . .   Address: . . . .

FORM 5

CONSENT FORM FOR EXPERIMENTAL PROCEDURE

Informed Consent for Studies of Exchange
Transfusion of Newborn Infants

I, mother . . . . . . or father . . . . . . of baby . . . . . . consent that an exchange transfusion can be performed by Dr. . . . . . on my baby for purposes of . . . . Dr. . . . . . explained to me that the procedure consists of replacing the baby's blood with that of a donor's blood following typing and cross-matching. The blood is exchanged by taking blood from . . . . . while reinfusing new blood through . . . . This procedure is known to be used for many diseases that newborn babies may have, and has been used for the last fifteen years by pediatricians. The risks of this method are very small, nevertheless, the doctor explained to me that the rare side effects reported are: mismatched blood, acidosis, low calcium level, infection, low temperature from cold blood. Under the circumstances in which this is to be done to my child, all known precautions to avoid or counteract these problems are being taken. The benefits expected by exchange transfusions would be an improvement in oxygen transport to all parts of the body.

I understand that this is an experimental procedure and that alternatives to this therapy are . . . . The information contained in this form has been verbally explained to me and all questions have been answered. I understand that I may withdraw my consent and discontinue the blood exchange transfusion at any time during the procedure and this will in no way jeopardize the continuing care of my child by the doctors assigned to his case.

Date   Signature of Parents

. . . .

Witnesses   . . . .

. . . .

. . . .

I certify that I have explained this procedure to the above mentioned parents and that they understand the contents of this consent. I will answer any inquiries concerning the blood transfusion during the procedure.

Signature of Doctor . . . .

point she attacked Harry Fried, a fourth-year medical student, when he failed to offer an adequate explanation of why babies with high bilirubin levels are given phototherapy: "Did you turn on the bili-lights without knowing the side effects? You should not believe anything is safe without thinking and asking. You should not trust anyone around here." In fact, throughout the month there was an ongoing debate as to when to put a baby under lights. The intern trained at Johns Hopkins was more conservative than the intern trained at University Hospital. The neonatology fellow believed in "waiting it out" where the data were questionable; the resident believed in "doing something."

An exchange transfusion represents one kind of experimentation. All services recognized the professional obligation not to submit a patient to the risks of an experimental measure unless there is nothing else to do, and even then, only with the consent of the patient. The clinical and moral perspectives overlap in the physician's decision to do an exchange transfusion. A second kind of experimentation is exemplified by the Clinical Research Center within University Hospital, which existed for the sole purpose of experimentation. For example, paid subjects would present themselves at the Clinical Research Center for clinical trials of new drugs for potential side effects. At no time did I witness the transfer of an in-house patient to the Clinical Research Center, though that does occur when more conventional therapies do not offer a sufficiently high probability of efficacy, or where the regular services are not equipped to handle a particular set of problems.

It is important to stress that the definition of *experimental,* compared to *innovative* or *acceptable* is a statement of relative placement on a medical range. Placement depends on both rational and nonrational factors determining the physician's judgment. It may depend on the setting in which he or she practices, the opinion of colleagues and associates, the frequency with which the physician uses the procedure, the familiarity of the physician with the relevant technical literature, and the availability of necessary facilities. On a more idiosyncratic basis, selection of an experimental therapy may depend on whether the physician likes to think of herself or himself as an innovator, the self-confidence of the physician in trying new techniques in the face of the more common acceptability of an alternative procedure, and assorted calendar pressures, such as available time, fatigue, and postprocedural schedule. The physician who is exhausted, overbooked, or about to take off on a vacation may opt for a conservative, widely accepted procedure over an experimental one.

Alan Cramer, an oncologist [cancer specialist] and the attending physician on general medical service, was leaving town for the weekend. He instructed his house officers that if Mary Scott, one of his private patients, came in during his absence, they should follow a plan of conservative management until his return on Monday morning. He explained that if he were not going out of town, he would recommend chemotherapy. The particular drug combination he advised was still controversial, and few physicians outside of university centers had even heard of it.

On a much more general level, students are continually faced with a need to explain the rational basis of their actions; consequently, they may have difficulty assimilating the nonrational as well as the rational explanations offered by superiors.

Medical students cite the textbook as justification for a recommendation for management. They are frequently taken aback by the response of the attending physician, who is likely to begin with the formulation, "Well, Harrison [textbook of internal medicine] may say that, but in my experience. . . . " For regardless of how the student excels at quoting the literature, he or she lacks the corroboration of personal experience. The house officer can cite personal experience but cannot use the phrase, "in my years of experience." It is commonplace for attending physicians to advise, "When you have seen as many . . . as I have, then you will be in a position to support your recommendation." But the invocation of personal experience is only one part of professional judgment within the medical perspective.

A second set of considerations arises from familiarity with the literature. One can marshal support from the literature in order to resolve an ambiguous situation. Where the evidence goes both ways, one can select arguments from the literature that suggest a trend in favor of doing x over doing y. One thus goes to the literature when one has limited personal experience. Finally, one makes use of the literature when one becomes sophisticated enough to realize that institutions as well as specialties have their biases, so that the institutional preference, such as that for electroconvulsive therapy, should not be assumed to be universal.

A third component is the availability of others to help make a difficult or unwanted decision. The distinction between difficult and easy decisions is affected by such factors as the stability of the patient's condition, the calculation of trade-offs (harm to the patient versus benefit, attenuation of one problem versus aggravation of another), the patient's age, the pressure of time, prognosis (will the procedure yield new information about which we can do something?), and the availability of alternatives (is there more than one procedure, drug, or treatment that can be tried with the same results?).

The hierarchical structure of the hospital bureaucracy makes available people of both higher and lower status who may contribute to the resolution of a clinical decision.[5] Whatever decisions a medical student is allowed to make must be supported by the supervising intern or resident. All student orders must be co-signed. While students will be given as much responsibility as they are capable of handling, they will always be protected by the house officer's legal responsibility. House officers use the attending physician or the private admitting physician when there is a hard decision to make that is outside the range of decisions with which they feel comfortable in assuming responsibility. The attending physician may feel it is necessary to get additional opinions from consulting services. For example, in the discussion about doing a tap, the opinion of the chief cardiologist was obtained, and it was used to bolster the recommendation of the attending physician. The system of referring decisions to someone with greater authority is known as "punting." When one depends on peers for their support and consultation, it is known as "covering." This occurs when one intern asks the other intern on the service to do a cardiac examination and to give an opinion on the need for further studies because "my ears for . . . defects are not so good."

An elderly physician told the following anecdote:

> An eminent physician was asked, "How do you make decisions?" He replied, "Based on my knowledge." He was then asked, "How did you get that knowledge?" To which he replied, "From my mistakes."

Within the medical perspective and its concern with concrete cases, specific references to the literature, individual experience, and judgment, there are sets of factors that can only be characterized as nonrational, which arise out of the fact that we are speaking of a human enterprise. Broadly speaking, the analysis of any data ultimately leads to the question, Do I feel comfortable with this course of action? Physicians vary in their willingness to take risks. They differ in their ability to learn from their mistakes. And even within the highly competitive university setting, some physicians rely more heavily on habit (customary choice) than do others. After discussing the program of patient management with the medical student, the resident asks, "Do you feel comfortable with it?" The attending physician responds, "This is what I feel comfortable doing." The experience of being "burned" makes everyone on a service more cautious, even when the discussion reveals a lack of rational grounding for the decision. For example, a fifty-five-year-old male patient, Smith, died from an unrecognized cardiac failure.

Resident: The night he came in I thought about putting him in the MICU. I thought about it with the EKG. He was sicker than he looked. I showed the EKG to three other people without giving them the history; they didn't suspect anything.

Attending physician: I think he should have gone to the MICU, though it's easy to say in retrospect.

Resident: Obviously, I can't disagree with you. Obviously he arrested and died.

The day following his death another patient was admitted to the service with a similar medical picture.

Attending physician: This is a guy with. . . . The better part of valor is to put him in the MICU and observe.

Resident: If you thought he had an MI [myocardial infarct, a heart attack] when he came in, this is three days out. He would have been coming out of the MICU the day we are putting him in.

Attending physician: I would watch him for a couple of days. Till we have a feel of which way his enzymes are going. He may be reinfarcting.

Resident: The problem is this . . . we're not even sure he's had an MI, even suspected MI, in a guy with a hemoglobin of 15. . . . He looks good and had no complaints. . . . If we put everyone in the MICU with. . . .

Attending physician: We made a mistake with Smith.

The ideal expressed by physicians with many years of experience that decision-making within the clinical perspective is something done as "second nature" on the basis of clinical evidence contrasts with the perplexity of the neophyte who occasionally wonders aloud at the long and convoluted process that is the embodiment of much medical decision-making. The debate may be lengthy, heated, and repetitive, but the ultimate decision is grounded in the clinical realities of the situation, expressed through history-taking, examination, diagnostic procedures, consultations, and the application of human judgment. The tendency to refer to patients by the complaints for which they were admitted ("the gall bladder") is nothing more than the tangible expression of this tendency to treat disease entities rather than people. This is so despite the fact that each patient has a unique constellation of problems, mediated by the particular skills and judgment of an individual physician. This reality contributes to the impossibility of a uniform standard of performance on the part of practitioners.

While the medical student is continually counseled to learn the mechanisms of pathology rather than particular treatments, so that he can accommodate himself to changes in medical technique and philosophy of treatment, the ultimate emphasis is on the specifications on each problem list. At the front of the record of each hospital admission is a listing of all the medical problems found in history-taking and examination.

The course of professional socialization is increasing familiarity with limitation, and the medical perspective requires the recognition of a variety of limits: the limitations of the individual practitioner in regard to both clinical knowledge and clinical skills; the limits of the disease entity (can sign a be attributed to disease b?); the limits of an individual case as a generalizable principle (how representative is this clinical picture of the classical description?); the limits of the current state of the art; and the limits of available institutional resources. In a most general sense, the use of the clinical perspective is a limitation on professional vision, the selection of a small segment of all possible considerations as the basis of physician insight. Physicians like to talk about the specialized form of thinking they begin to learn as they undertake their professional training. But professional identity also entails learning a particular mode of seeing—removing some blinders and acquiring others. The student physician learns to read meaning from a patient's shuffling gait, when even the patient is not aware of how he looks when walking. Yet the student physician can also learn to become unaware of the visible signs of social discrimination which surround him or her within the hospital organization. The identification of a clinical perspective is a way of saying that within professional training, and with the acquisition of social status in a complex social organization, one learns to "see" a limited realm of things as problems, as well as a limited range of solutions to those problems.

6 The Legal Perspective

Increasingly we find ourselves turning to the courts to render judgments about the complexities of medical practice, particularly as they impinge upon questions of the quality of life that individuals may enjoy. Implicitly, we ask the courts to arbitrate between the moral claims of the physician and those of the layperson, though we disguise the issue of competing moral claims by applying the more neutral labels of defendant and plaintiff. With confidence in the capacity of the law and its agents in the legal profession, we appeal to the courts for a "right to die" or for compensation for damages suffered through alleged "malpractice." This confidence in the wisdom of the law and its servants ignores the peculiar relationship with the law that physicians have typically enjoyed. In this chapter a rather technical set of arguments will be made to depict the limits we should place on that confidence. Specifically, physicians have been until recently the main actors in the judicial process intended to constrain their actions. By introducing standards of "expert testimony" and of "community practice," the courts have guaranteed physicians substantive protection from charges of incompetence.

What follows is a preliminary description of the legal process, analogous to the range of clinical practice. Informed consent is offered as an example of the creative process within the law. As the idea of informed consent has matured, it has led to a shift away from the legal notion of community standards of medical practice toward a standard of judgment predicated on what a "reasonable" patient would expect to know. This is a significant development because it diminishes physician autonomy while augmenting patient participation and responsibility in clinical decisions.

The identification of a problem within the legal perspective evokes a process of problem-solving comparable to that of medicine. Any discussion of the legal process is a depiction of the development of legal principle,[1] starting with the search for historical precedents and evolving through the introduction of legal principle, acceptance into the legal canon, modification, and possible departure from the legal corpus (post-principle).[2] The concept of informed consent will be used to demonstrate the evolution of the legal process.

Informed consent came into its own as a doctrine of law in the early 1960s[3] with *Natanson* v. *Kline* (1960). Earlier rulings which contributed to its establishment include *Pratt* v. *Davis* (1905), *Barnett* v. *Bachrach* (1943), and *Bang* v. *Charles T. Miller Hospital* (1955).[4]

In *Natanson* v. *Kline,* the court ruled that neither a physician nor a surgeon may

> violate without permission the bodily integrity of his patient by a major or capital operation, placing him under an anaesthetic for that purpose and operating on him without his consent or knowledge.[5]

The doctrine of informed consent is grounded in theories of battery or negligence.[6] Regardless of which theoretical basis is preferred, the significant requirements of informed consent are that the patient must be aware of the risks involved in accepting treatment, and the patient must agree to the treatment.[7] The patient-physician relationship, as a fiduciary relationship, requires that the physician ensure that awareness and assent exist before proceeding with treatment.[8] Even when the patient consents to the procedure and its related risks, it does not relieve the doctor of liability for negligence occurring in the course of treatment.[9]

The issue of disclosing risks is of particular concern, for it is here that interpretation of the law has gradually changed. The issue is one of scope. Must a physician reveal all collateral risks? As Waltz and Scheuneman point out, a distinction must be made between the risks a physician *could* disclose and those he *should* disclose. Obviously a physician cannot disclose risks about which he or she is uninformed; consequently, physicians have an obligation to be informed of the risks entailed in a given procedure or drug. Taken one step further, this touches on risks that are known to others in the profession as well as the need to investigate risks that are as yet unknown. This latter step invokes the range of the medical perspective, with its distinctions between experimental and customary practice. It is evident that the theoretical underpinning of negligence is a part of this issue, even in situations where patients have agreed to the ensuing "touching,"* based on their understanding of revealed risks.

The location of medical practice on this range will vary with regard to who makes the evaluation, for what period of time, and with respect to what population of patients. The physician practicing in the university teaching hospital is likely to consider a practice customary before a rural practitioner. Similarly, within a five-year period, procedure x may be customary within academic medicine, innovative among urban local practitioners, and experimental among physicians practicing in a rural setting. Third, physicians may vary in their willingness to take risks, depending on the likelihood of morbidity, the absence of restraining opinion (for example, "chief's cases," which have no private physicians), and the financial resources of the patient for the procurement of scarce, expensive drugs or equipment. With the notion of "standards of practice," the law touches on these variables without spelling them out.

A physician need not disclose all possible risks, and clearly something less than total disclosure will satisfy the law. The numerous cases that have pertained to this issue use the formula of community practice, according to which the physician is obligated to act in accordance with the custom and practice of physicians within the "community."[10] At times this has meant "what a reasonable physician would do under the circumstances";[11] at other times it has meant that disclosure must be consistent with "good medical practice."[12] This argument rests on the concept of "standardization" and requires the test of "expert" testimony.[13]

Before turning to the community practice argument, it is necessary to know what limits physician disclosure. A primary limitation is the notion of "therapeutic privilege."[14] If, in the physician's judgment, disclosure of collateral risks will be too upsetting to the patient, based on his or her familiarity with the patient, the physician may withhold the information. For example, the physician may argue that the emotional disturbance created by the need for surgery may make the patient unable to respond to a 10 percent chance of postsurgical

---

*In the law, "touching" means allowing another person to violate the common rules of bodily privacy.

complications without using that risk as a condition of refusing surgery; therefore, the physician does not inform the patient of that risk. Obviously there is difficulty in evaluating the counterclaim of the patient, ex post facto, that he or she was capable of absorbing the emotional burden of the disclosure of material risks and that if he or she had known of these risks, consent would have been withheld. Of course, as long as those risks fail to materialize there is no problem. Regardless of whether the physician's estimation of the patient's capacity to absorb information about collateral risks was correct, there remains the substitution of the physician's judgment of the patient's well-being for the patient's self-determination.

The community practice argument goes hand in hand with therapeutic privilege. The latter is grounded in the assumption that physicians, because of their membership in a professional group with the protected status of experts, can make certain claims to knowledge outside the ken of their clients which is acquired through their extensive professional education.[15] This allows them the prerogative of "protecting" their clients from possible harm. Thus, the law identifies *community* with the community of physicians rather than the community of patients.

Problems have arisen when there is a need to validate these assumptions in order to determine professional negligence with regard to failure to disclose risks. The practice has been to solicit testimony from expert witnesses, other physicians practicing in the same or similar communities who might clarify whether the named physician has acted in accordance with professional standards.[16] Because physicians are generally unwilling to testify against each other, the use of community standards as a determinant of informed consent is of limited value.[17] Second, the idea of community practice creates the possibility that if enough physicians in a community practice a substandard form of medicine but are willing to testify to its "normality," charges of negligence would be difficult to prove.[18] This danger suggests the need for periodic recertification of physicians in order to ensure that they maintain a level of skill which could be evaluated as meeting community standards of professional proficiency.

Eleanor Glass argues for the restructuring of informed consent. She stresses that therapeutic privilege denies the patient the right to say yes to treatment. She asks how the patient can be protected from the physician's use of privilege to manipulate both the patient and the situation, even though the law looks askance at physicians who manipulate information in order to get the patient's consent.[19]

"Overselling" is the deliberate withholding of frightening information from the patient.[20] Physicians may also manipulate their patients into compliance by threatening the termination of the fiduciary relationship, the substitution of less desirable forms of treatment for the recommended one, and suspension of available treatment if the patient fails to meet the recommended time limit for accepting treatment. Physicians may go so far as to offer misleading or outright false representations of the nature of the problem in order to offer a "story" that will conform to the patient's own need for an explanation. For example, if it is known that the patient thinks the problem is his heart, even when that belief is unfounded, the physician may offer such an explanation to get the patient to accept the proposed plan of treatment.

In contrast to the "'reasonable' doctor standard," Glass introduces the "patient's standard of care" argument.[21] The jury, instead of placing itself "in the shoes of the physician," is asked to envision itself as the patient; it is then asked to decide as another layperson the relevance of the information that was withheld from the patient. While previously testimony depended on "what must a 'reasonable' physician do in order to obtain informed consent, Glass entertains employing a standard which favors the patient's judgment and expectations. Rather than requiring an expert schooled in the intricacies of medical jurisprudence, this argument contends that laypersons can evaluate the salient issues and testimony. Furthermore, it negates the assumption that only physicians can judge the standards of practice within the community. Though by Glass's account there was little support for her argument at the time of publication, this is the direction in which the law pertaining to informed consent is now moving.[22]

Expert testimony, whether from ballistics experts or pathologists, is provided for the benefit of the jury, but it is not binding. The utilization of the patient's standard of care is an application of this principle, and to that extent it is unremarkable. In the past, when experts have given conflicting testimony, it has fallen to the jury to decide the relative merit of the opposing arguments. What is noteworthy, however, is that this standard removes the need for expert testimony, as it throws the burden to disclose material risks on the physician as judged by the community of patient-peers and not by the community of physician-peers. It thus recognizes the vulnerability of standardization and the encumbent problems of expanding the domain of "the community" furthermore, it acknowledges that the position of the patient is distinct from that of the physician and is not just a matter of more limited knowledge. It is the patient who is subject to potential risks; it is he or she who suffers from inappropriate protection, from inadequate or overwhelming disclosure.

A series of recent legal decisions illustrates this shift in emphasis (table 4). Several commentators have noted that changes in the standards for informed consent improve the patient-physician relationship by increasing communication between the two parties and increasing patient autonomy, without reducing the quality of medicine being practiced.[23] Despite the unproven fears that the substitution of the reasonable patient standard for the community practice standard would elicit a volume of malpractice litigation that would have been impossible under the old standard, the more common argument has been similar to the following conclusion:

> *Trogun v. Fruchtman* stands out as having the greatest potential for furthering patients' interests by promoting greater doctor-patient communication, thereby lessening the chance that malpractice action will be brought.[24]

From the introduction of informed consent as a legal doctrine in the early 1960s and its acceptance into the legal canon, we have seen the gradual change in its enactment without the overturning of its underlying principles of awareness and assent. Subsequent modifications are likely to occur, expanding on the needs of the "reasonable patient." What has been suggested is that the law, like the medical perspective, deals with case-by-case review of a problem, selecting and applying appropriate principles to the unique situation of each case. Second, it attempts to circumscribe general problems by dealing in concrete terms, matters of fact, rather than subjective criteria. In doing so, it has tended to utilize "expert testimony," "community practice," and "therapeutic privilege" as means of locating the relevant criteria in the hands of a recognizable group of people with similar training and professional experience. At the same time the courts, as agents of the law, have become aware of the limitations of such practice vis à vis the interests of the patient. The trend has been to relocate the burden of judgment in the jury, where the standards of the layperson take precedent over any presentation of expert testimony; in

TABLE 4

Landmark Cases in the Development of "Patient's Standard of Care" Argument

1914   *Schloendorff* v. *Society of New York Hospital*

Establishes battery as theory of recovery for liability. Negates need for establishing standard of practice within the community (211 N.Y. 125, 105 N.E. 92 [1914]).

1971   *Cooper* v. *Roberts*

Overturns "reasonable physician standard." Declares duty of physician to disclose material risks based on fiduciary relationship and not based on standard practice in physician's community. Court recognized so-called "conspiracy of silence" as preventing effective physician testimony (220 Pa. Sup. 260, 286 A.2d 676, 689 [1972]).

1972   *Wilkinson* v. *Vesey*

Establishes that patient must be given all material information necessary to make a judgment. Introduces "what a 'reasonable' person must know" as test of materiality (110 R.I. 609, 629, 295 A.2d 676, 689 [1972]).

1972   *Cobbs* v. *Grant*

Declares that patient must be informed of known risks of death or serious bodily harm using test of "what the patient needs to know" (8 Cal.3d 229, 502 P. 1, 104 Cal Reptr. 505 [1972]).

1973   *Roe* v. *Wade*

The so-called "abortion ruling" establishes the right of women to obtain first-trimester abortions and, with limitations, second-trimester abortions. Informed consent is considered as part of the "right to privacy" with recognition that it enhances patient autonomy (410 U.S. 113 [1973]).

fact, there need be no presentation of experts. The legal process carries within itself a movement from the specific to the general, with the possibility that when a legal principle becomes too broad it becomes meaningless and is replaced by the citation of a new, more highly circumscribed principle.

The general theories of assault and negligence have been noted as the sources of the doctrine of informed consent. The early rulings dealt with the specific concerns of unlawful touching and negligence on the basis of the community practice standard. With the adaptation of the law to the additional problems of emergencies, disclosure of risks, and the meaning of "locality," the courts broadened the scope of informed consent to include the dependence of the patient on the physician's fulfillment of the fiduciary relationship. In so doing, the courts have succeeded in expanding the rights of the patient, and this will probably affect the nature of medical practice.

But practical considerations remain, particularly the feasibility of fulfilling the legal requirements of informed consent within the everyday world of clinical practice. The first obstacle is one of time. Can physicians afford the time to disclose the material information necessary for a patient's decision to accept or reject treatment, when the volume of patients determines income in a fee-for-service practice? The second obstacle is the continuum of medical procedures for which informed consent is required. Very few physicians would argue that they must get the express consent of patients to do a venipuncture, and all would respect the need for informed consent in a nonemergency appendectomy; but the bulk of medical practice falls somewhere in-between. The third obstacle is the public-private dimension of medical practice. As the problems inherent in therapeutic privilege illustrate, changes in the nature of informed consent occur with changes in the visibility of medical practice. Where a "conspiracy of silence" on the part of physicians is a source of protection, there is greater latitude for "professional behavior." Informed consent as a possible source of malpractice litigation becomes increasingly relevant to the practitioner who believes that his work may become public because of his patient's awareness of the possibility of bringing suit, because of the greater feasibility of documentation through the presence of observers, and because of the unavailability of peer support through the exclusion of professional standards as the sole determinant of negligence.[25]

From the clinical perspective, informed consent can only be an approximation. From the legal perspective, it is only workable if the burden of litigation does not become so great as to clog the machinery of the courts. It is tenable only as long as the fear of malpractice suits does not create inferior medical care, based on undue caution and inflated expense. To the extent that the patient-physician relationship is a fiduciary one, there is an intrinsic limit to the autonomy of the patient. The question remains, At what point is that relationship dissolved by the demands of patients for autonomy, which the physician finds detrimental to the execution of his professional obligations? In part, this is the question of what justifies an emergency suspension of the need for consent.

Fear of malpractice charges may mean that physicians are slow to adopt innovative procedures out of fear of the risks of disclosure, so that patients are deprived of the benefit of new drugs and techniques which would otherwise be used. Also, patients may be subjected to unnecessary tests for the sake of "covering all bases," as protection against charges of negligence. On a rotation in psychiatry, an example of this phenomenon occurred:

> The resident requested from the fourth-year student spinal films on a woman who was a candidate for ECT (shock treatments). The fourth-year student thought films were being obtained because the resident wanted to identify the source of her back pain. The resident in fact wanted to document any existing hairline breaks or abnormalities of the spine, so that the patient could not later bring suit based on the harmful effects of ECT. (If the muscle relaxant and anesthesia are improperly administered, the stress on the body from the electric shock can break bones.) The student was told that if he thought the patient would agree to the films on the pretense of diagnosing her back pain, he should secure her consent on that basis.

Despite the difficulties inherent in the consistent and substantive practice of obtaining informed consent, there are reasons for its survival. It is a legal principle that must be subscribed to for the sake of physician integrity and patient autonomy. It reinforces professional standards of practice, while at the same time it draws the patient into the decision-making process. This basis for mutual exchange and support is likely to minimize dissatisfaction on the part of both parties and thus, in the long run, contribute to better health care. But this optimism leads into the ongoing debate on whether the courts can be the cutting edge of change: can the courts precipitate changes in legislation and ultimately, through moral suasion, modify individuals' values and beliefs? Certainly the creation of informed consent is only the first step in the evolution of a social change.

Many physicians still have to be won over to the value of informed consent, because they see it as a bookkeeping chore developed by the hospital bureaucracy; sometimes they may treat it as institutionalized distrust of their clinical judgment. Likewise, the day-to-day meaning of informed consent remains mysterious to many patients, who still feel obligated to sign whatever slips of paper are put before them. After all, a state of illness or malaise is not conducive to aggressive behavior. Moreover, most patients are too insecure in their own sense of competence, to push the physician for further explanation or elaboration.

The vast changes in the practice of medicine in the last two decades have increased the salience of the legal perspective in clinical practice, while evoking the need to pay increasing attention to the moral perspective. The first effect is a consequence of the increasing incidence of malpractice litigation, the rising costs of malpractice awards to plaintiffs, the passage of "good samaritan" laws, and the eagerness of the media to publicize medical-legal issues. All of these factors have led to increasing consciousness of legal vulnerability on the part of physicians. Medical students report that legal information is incorporated into classroom lectures on the recognition and treatment of disorders which have potential for legal problems. In cases of head trauma and a possible "missed" concussion, for example, students are cautioned to secure skull x-rays regardless of the apparent seriousness of the injury. The visibility of ethical issues within medicine is heightened by the media, including films and novels. *One Flew Over the Cuckoo's Nest* comes to mind, as well as *Bang the Drum Slowly,* both as movies and as books. As an increasingly large portion of health care is delegated to physicians in the hospital setting, technological bases of medicine become the mainstay of medical care. With the acceptance of technology, both physicians and patients find problems that were unknown in pretechnological eras.

The increasing salience of the legal perspective and the increasing relevance of the moral perspective contribute to the classic biases of the field of medicine. As Thomas Scheff puts it, when in doubt, diagnose illness.[26] Even though it is just as much an error to pronounce a well person "sick," this error is seen as more tolerable than calling a sick person well. The juncture between the legal and clinical perspectives is also characterized by this bias toward overtreatment. Fears of legal suits persuade physicians to get needless x-rays, while the presence of sophisticated equipment tempts physicians to use it rather than let it go to waste.

In considering both the medical and legal perspectives as perspectives on problem-solving, we have seen that each is wedded to case-by-case review, logical argument. Each restricts its concept of generalization. Even though each case may be similar to other cases with its general attributes, the focus of argumentation is on factors which make the case dissimilar or unique. Sometimes this takes the form of saying: "Since we've failed to find dissimilarities in this situation, we can treat it as a 'classic' case." The perspectives differ in the scope of their respective concerns, however. The medical perspective is grounded in body systems. It demands that the physician employ the senses in the service of reasoning and organization of date.[27] The test of the validity of professional judgment is the patient's recovery or improvement, as opposed to the patient's deterioration or death. Finally, it has been suggested that the clinical perspective is affected by transformations of private medical practice into situations of public performance.

The legal perspective goes beyond the concretized case, back into the legal corpus to select relevant precedents and forward to propose modifications in the law. The lawyer's test of the validity of professional judgment is broader than the physician's. It may encompass a longer period than a human lifetime. It may go unrecognized until some later court cites the opinion as relevant to a current problem. More important, law deals with concepts such as "liberty" and "privacy," which are subject to greater vagaries than are anatomical landmarks.

7 The Moral Perspective

The progression of this analysis, from the clinical perspective through the legal perspective and on to the moral perspective, is characteristic of how physicians resolve ethical issues in the clinical setting. It is not always necessary or practical to complete the progression, and some physicians never venture beyond the legal perspective. Sometimes the boundaries between perspectives are not so clear as these arguments would imply; however, to treat them as discrete categories of understanding is a heuristic device.

From the sociologist's vantage point, analysis of moral arguments entails the description of both epistemological and social considerations. In very broad terms we are asking: How do we know what we know? What can we know? and What do we know? Much of the time we take for granted what we know to be "moral," even though it is culturally relative to our membership in particular social categories. The moral code of an urban street gang is distinct from that of a white-collar executive. Over time the definition of *the moral* may also change, so that behavior that was "immoral" for our parents may be permissible for ourselves. Therefore, knowledge of what is moral is a part of social dynamics that is affected by time, place, and the identity of the actors.

In contrasting the law and morality, Alexander Capron states, "Law and morality are similar in that both attempt to prescribe human behavior according to a set of rights and duties." In the course of his arguments he develops the significant differences between the two, which are derived from a discussion of rights and which support the hypothesis that "there is no necessary connection between law and morality." This entails a rejection of two claims: that the law is a codification of morals, and that law takes the place of morals. The first claim he dismisses as a syllogism: "Since the people create the law and the people hold moral views, therefore the law enacts morality." The second, he argues, belies the actual condition of fact. Law is instituted when the moral system fails to function. He distinguishes between law and morality in the following ways:

> First, the heart of a moral system is its judgments of right and wrong in an outward-referring sense, while the heart of the legal system is the ordering of relationships, in which only rules of consistency with the system's own rules need be sought.
>
> A second difference arises from this matter of "reference." If you found yourself alone on the proverbial desert island, you might find cause to employ a moral system, but you would have no use in any reasonable sense for a legal system. If, however, I were then to be washed ashore on your island, a need for laws would arise.[1]

The practical effect of these distinctions is that one may criticize a law as being "unjust" and introduce a moral claim for its repudiation; however, the claim does not attain the binding force of law as it is not recognized as being legitimately founded in the law. As long as the law provides physicians with the "therapeutic privilege" to withhold information from a patient, one can exhort them to do otherwise as moral human beings, but it does not change the law. Neither morality nor law carries within it the assurance that the named obligations will be fulfilled.

Like the other two perspectives, the moral perspective has its range of change. With regard to social behavior, one can characterize a range from moral proscription through prescription, with points of disapproval, toleration, and acceptance between the poles. For example, a proscription such as "thou shalt not kill" can shift to disapproval ("thou shalt not kill except as a last resort in self-defense"), toleration ("thou may kill to protect thy life or property"), acceptance ("thou may kill to protect thy country"), and prescription ("thou shall kill thy enemies"). But unlike the ranges common to the medical and the legal perspectives, the moral perspective may turn back upon itself. That is, a behavior which has moved from proscription to prescription may gradually return to the category of taboo behavior, as, for example, the prescription "thou shall kill one's enemies" may in peacetime revert to some milder claim.

Examples of change within the moral perspective are so numerous as to suggest that there is no "morality" per se, only the evocation of moral questions within specific situations. Thus, we may speak of ethical relativism, or its expression in "situational ethics."[2] Within the clinical setting there is a bias in favor of this mode of moral analysis, though it rarely contributes to the development of systematic moral judgment. The reasons for this will now be developed.

Questions of value and belief are traditionally matters for philosophers and theologians to ponder; however, sociologists also concern themselves with these questions, asking how values and beliefs are acquired, maintained, and changed.[3] Since sociologists are more concerned with the process by which values and beliefs are integrated into daily life, they are likely to appear evasive about defining what is "good, desirable, or right." I shall leave the burden of clarification to experts in moral philosophy, for I do not wish to imply that I possess such expertise.[4] I do want, however, to clarify the meaning of "a moral perspective" as it has been used in the previous discussion.

In looking at the language of moral philosophy, we can identify some of the problems that arise when we try to determine whether or not physicians make "moral judgments." Broadly speaking, we are talking about a process of generalization in which disparate actions are compared and found to have a common identity as "obligatory, right or wrong, good or bad, permissible or forbidden."[5] These generalizations also serve the purpose of identifying situations which evoke the need to modify existing moral rules or to create new ones. Sometimes this means identifying an entirely different set of moral rules as appropriate to the situation. For example, Mr. Jones has just been diagnosed as having cancer of the esophagus. The second-year medical student says, "Every patient ought to be told the truth." His implied reason is that truthfulness is both desirable and obligatory behavior for physicians.[6] In contrast, the attending physician replies, "Only some patients want to hear the truth, and it is your responsibility to protect the patient from unnecessary trauma, which might preclude his compliance with a required regimen." This can be translated as, "Professional behavior demands paternalism."[7] As part of the student's socialization he or she learns to appreciate the moral rules pertaining to paternalism, as other considerations become less salient. While philosophers continually talk about individuals and the moral rules they apply, sociologists emphasize how the adoption of these principles is a function of group membership, often stressing how the group helps create the moral concerns that are subsequently treated as external to the group.[8]

We have seen repeatedly that medical students may be instructed by the attending physician in how to deal with a specific situation, for example, whether Baby Boy Jones should be given phototherapy for neonatal jaundice; but they rarely present any general moral principles as the underpinnings of that "right action." Instead, the proposition is converted into the language of clinical judgment, with the evaluation of whether the treatment is "appropriate" and the subsequent identification of "the treatment of choice." In the substitution of *appropriate* for *right* we find constraints against defining the evaluative process as intrinsically moral. Moreover, since the "right action" is so closely bounded by the specifics of this particular clinical instance, discussion can be extensive without uncovering any general moral principles. Clinical judgment, with its prerequisites of prolonged education, personal experience, and institutionalized consultation, obfuscates the possibility that this particular case may demonstrate some generalizable moral concept, such as obligation. Medical students are rarely asked to take cases A, B, C, and D, for example, and relate them to a more generalizable case; instead, they are taught that each case is "unique and special" in its particular dimensions. Therefore, it is important to realize that while a situation may be converted to a moral framework, from the perspective of the physician and medical student it is a clinical problem and not a moral one. Furthermore, to appraise the situation as one of subconscious morality, which legitimates the assumption of a moral grounding for all clinical behavior, ignores how the decision-making process is interpreted by its own practitioners.

In formal philosophical terms, moral philosophers talk to two categories of ethical theories. Deontological (formalist) theory holds that the rightness or wrongness of an action is determined by identifying the kind of action or its intention. What matters in the determination of "rightness" is the nature of the action or the reason for performing it, and not its outcome. Teleological (consequentialist) theory holds that the rightness or wrongness of an action is determined by its outcome. Sociologists are more likely to talk about means-and-end relationships: whether we should judge the rightness of an action by the desirability of the means employed, or by the end achieved, or by some combination of these considerations.[9] Indeed, within the medical sphere, we find a curious blending of both formalist and consequentialist thinking, so that neither category, taken alone, seems wholly satisfactory.

The extensive discussion of the meaning of the phrase, "First, do no harm," from the Hippocratic oath, has gradually blurred the distinction between intention and outcome, as in the doctrine of double effect.[10] Some actions have both good and bad consequences as their inevitable outcome. Such an action is permissible, and the bad consequence is morally permissible, if certain conditions are met.[11] The doctrine of double effect is frequently applied to the prescription of opiate painkillers in the case of terminally ill patients as well as to the situation of abortion.[12] The locus of the moral rules in such instances varies from the physician's intention to the evaluation of probable outcome without being solely deontological or teleological in formulation.

Again, clinical discussion is not based on deontological and teleological considerations, even though these distinctions may be teased out of clinical practice. For example, in the event of an unexpected death as a result of surgery, physicians express a variety of feelings including anger, chagrin, sadness, and denial. However, they are not likely to convert the death into an example of deontological principle such as, "Killing is bad, but if the intention of the surgeon was to extend a life, then the unexpected outcome of death is not morally indefensible." The same situation can be converted to a teleological dictum: "Surgeons are obligated to 'save' the patients 'medicine men' give up on; when they fail, they are morally culpable." This is yet another way of showing that physicians act within multiple moral universes, with principles that are selectively evoked within highly circumscribed social environments. It is a matter not of "a moral system" but of "moral systems."

Human socialization reveals the development of moral systems. All of us start out in life with the moral precepts parents provide, implicitly if not explicitly.[13] As small children we are often introduced to formal systems of religious belief which enrich our notions of right and wrong. As we grow older, particularly in that phase of adolescence known as "the identity crisis," we test the validity of these principles, often discarding what seems unsatisfactory. In adulthood we may practice a profession which also provides normative ethical concerns, though these tend to be applied on fairly circumscribed occasions. Yet sometimes, in professional performance, these more recently acquired rules fail us. They appear inapplicable or inappropriate, or situational factors create within us an ambivalence which asks us to choose among professional morals, civic morals, (those rules pertaining to our membership in the polity), and what I would call personal morals.

It could be argued that individuals do not negate, deny, or in any way repudiate their personal systems of morals when they refer to standards of action predicated on professional membership or the law. For the most part, this is true. But there are times, particularly in the case of medical students, when people do not reach back into their personal systems of morals to make clear their allegiance to a model of professional action to which they aspire. In time, they cease to consider the appropriateness of looking back to that earlier system of normative principles.

As has been stated before, the systems of values identified from these three vantage points are frequently consistent with one another, necessitating no acknowledgment of their mutuality. Only in situations of conflict does the medical student or physician become aware that these sources of rightness and wrongness are in disagreement, both in their determination of what is "the right thing to do" and, conceivably, in their outcome. It is at this point of disagreement that physicians are likely to talk about the practice of medicine as "a whole other way of thinking."

Having exhausted their clinical options to reverse or to stabilize a life-threatening condition physicians employ a model of decision-making which looks like this: the contributions of clinical expertise through medication or procedures to support the patient throughout the process of inevitable deterioration, which advances to the relevance of existing legal considerations to avoid medical negligence or malpractice, and then concludes with the search for standards of action founded on personal values and beliefs which might allow the physician to act upon a standard of personal care, defined by physicians as "what I would want done if the patient were my parent, my spouse, or my sibling."

Though greatly oversimplified, this is a movement from a teleological schema to a deontological one, corresponding to a movement from a system of professional morals to one of personal morals. But

these distinctions are less clear in practice because physicians subscribe to the fictitious notion that they treat all patients in universalistic
terms.[14] It has been the task of medical sociologists to demonstrate
why and how this fails as a description of professional practice.[15]
Thus, in the process of elaboration we find that the supposition of "one
ethical system" is also fallacious; hence, the adoption of three
nomenclatures—the clinical, the legal, and the moral perspectives.

The following situations demonstrate the evocation of either
the legal or the moral perspective in conjunction with the preexisting
clinical perspective. They help to demonstrate how uncertainty and
ambiguity are resolved by the use of the professional style of decision-making, which originates with the clinical perspective.

> A young woman comes into the emergency room, reports she has
> recently returned from the Yucatan, and complains of symptons
> that seem to fit a description of either malaria or typhoid fever. It is
> late at night, and she is offered admission the next morning. She is
> very ambivalent about coming into the hospital. She asks, "Will
> anything happen to me if I don't show?" The examining physician
> replies, "Well, we'll send the police to get you, and they are
> required to take you to City Hospital [a public hospital known for
> its horror tales]." The woman returns to University Hospital the
> next day. (clinical, legal perspectives; no moral perspective)

> A forty-six-year-old woman has had repeated hospitalizations for
> a fever of unknown origins. She has undergone numerous tests
> which failed to reveal the source of her fever. She has never had a
> pelvic examination and refuses to agree to one, as she believes it
> inappropriate to her maiden status. While everyone concerned
> with her care is certain that this must be done, they refrain because
> "an unauthorized pelvic is r-a-p-e." (clinical, legal perspectives;
> latent moral perspective)

> The pulmonary attending physician discusses the management of
> viral pneumonia in a patient with a known neurological deficit.
> "We know we can probably get him over the acute episode . . . but
> we've not dealt with the basic problem—what do we do from here?
> He's demented. Once you get him over this episode you will be
> saving him for the next." Meanwhile the consulting neurologist is
> urging the team to "press on." (clinical, moral perspectives; no
> legal perspective)

In practice there are three distinct orderings of relevant perspectives for the physician: (1) the clinical, the legal, and the moral; (2) the clinical, the moral, and the legal; and (3) the clinical, without either the legal or the moral.

The case of a child who suffered from kidney failure exemplifies the first category. No kidney donor was available and the mother's religion (Jehovah's Witness) would have made a transplant unacceptable in any case.[16] The child's case was presented to the chief of the renal section, the legal responsibilities were reviewed, and the situation was ultimately resolved on moral grounds; however, the actors were likely to characterize their decision as based on the clinical grounds that they had "nothing to offer him." The decision was made to allow the child to die from kidney shutdown, rather than extend his suffering through dialysis on a crisis basis. Since the patient was only nine years old, no program would accept him for chronic dialysis, and without the prospect of transplant surgery such stopgap measures would have been pointless. Yet a purely clinical solution would have involved repeated efforts to gain the child another month—or week or day—of life. Since there was no treatment to offer the patient, there was no possibility of legal maneuvering. With the acceptance of the mother's religious beliefs as rational, the issue was resolved in favor of supporting her in her decision, that is, using a moral perspective.

The second category of ordering is more rare, but it is exemplified in the much publicized Quinlan case. Without the clinical picture of "a vegetative state," the moral and legal issues would not arise. To the extent that Karen Ann Quinlan's physicians believed there were medical options to offer her, the case remained a medical problem. Without the support of their parish priest, who indicated the position of the Catholic church in these matters (the church argues that medical heroics may cease when there is no hope of recovery), the parents would never have challenged their physicians. Second, without their confidence in the moral correctness of their plea for minimal support, they would not have moved the physicians and the governing hospital to consider the legal ramifications of the case. In medical practice this is not really an exceptional case, and informal institutional mechanisms would normally prevail. This time, however, the media picked up the issues, and the case became a *cause célèbre*. The public interest in the moral issues contributed little to a concrete solution of a complex problem, and the legal opinion of the court provided little genuine clarification. Its chief effect is to warn physicians that when their private actions come into public view, they are liable for the consequences of their actions. The difficulty of the Quinlan family in finding a hospital or nursing home to accept their daughter and to allow her to die is predicated on the fear of legal action against the medical institution in the event of her death. The fear of charges of criminal negligence exists, regardless of the moral sentiment of the laity. But without the widespread belief in a right to die, the courts would not be used to clarify a moral ethos. While the ranking is not so clear as it might be, it does suggest the murky boundaries between perspectives and the difficulty in assigning ascendancy to one or another.

The third category is the most common, and numerous examples have already been cited. The clinical perspective is dominant in the clinical setting. Where it is adequate to existing problems, no attempt is made to move past it in order to examine latent moral or legal issues.

It would seem that there are two other general formulations of ranking with regard to these competing perspectives. For the hospital administration, the ranking is legal, medical, and moral. Often, for the patient or layperson, it is moral, medical, and legal. The moral perspective may be identified with personal judgment; the medical arises in consultation with the physician; the legal is introduced when the patient has failed to profit from the first two perspectives. Independent of the advice of professionally trained experts, the only basis for problem-solving for the patient or layperson is a moral stance: What is the right thing for me to do? Where the patient and the physician differ as to what is best for the patient, a third opinion may be sought, perhaps from the hospital administrator, as is the case when the patient wishes to sign out "against medical advice" or to refuse offered treatment (see form 3). This frequently marks the collision course of the three competing perspectives.

By returning to the case of the nine-year-old child of the Jehovah's Witness, we can summarize the use of the clinical, legal, and ethical perspectives. The child, a boy, was admitted for treatment of exacerbated kidney failure. His condition warranted consideration of transfusion and dialysis. His chart was stamped "Jehovah's Witness." Because the child needed a transplantation of a donor kidney, orders were given from the renal service to hold off transfusing him until the situation was critical (a blood transfusion would affect the antibodies in his blood, which might be detrimental to his body's acceptance of foreign tissue). Since it was already 9 P.M., the decision was made to hold the patient till morning, when a decision on dialysis could be made by the full complement of staff. This was the night of the house staff's annual party. The third-year medical student spent the night doing routine work and writing up the case.

While the student was initially in favor of sending the child out on peritoneal dialysis (dialysis through the abdominal cavity) the hospital director believed that the mother should be supported in her decision to refuse transfusions and transplantation of a donor kidney, because to him it appeared that she was quite rational. He stated that he does not recommend chronic dialysis without consent for a kidney transplant when a donor kidney becomes available, because it is ultimately unfair to the child. Though legal intervention was possible, he was not anxious to go to court because, he argued, "We have nothing to offer the child." There was no available kidney donor within the family; the father was dead and the siblings were all minors, considerably younger than the patient. There was no possibility of placing him in a program for chronic dialysis, given his age.

The intern railed, "I'm really sick about it. It's his life that she has made a decision on." The third-year student was clearly upset. He repeatedly spoke of how "each of us has to challenge his beliefs according to his vision of God." Meanwhile, the mother insisted, "If he is going to die, let him die now without putting him through surgery. . . . Nothing—not blood or anything else—is going to determine whether he lives. What happens is God's will."

The child was given replacement fluids, which improved his electrolyte levels. He was dialyzed as a means of buying time to make a decision, and then sent home to die of uremic poisoning, which is a slow but relatively painless death.

Looking at the relevant perspectives of the mother, the hospital administrator, and the medical student and his supervising resident, we get the following rank orders: First, the mother based her arguments on her religious beliefs and made a credible claim that these were also the beliefs of her deceased husband and all her children. While she acknowledged the severity of her son's medical condition, she remained steadfast. The fact that she requested that her son's chart be stamped "Jehovah's Witness" illustrates some familiarity with the relevant legal arguments, but the mother discussed the legal considerations only when pushed by me or the administrator. My role as a sociologist was revealed to the mother, and the administrator encouraged me to ask whatever questions I wished. Second, the hospital administrator accepted the clinical report from the medical student but considered it his responsibility to weigh the possibility of calling up a cooperative judge and getting a court order for any needed transfusion. He evaluated the mother's arguments to ascertain that they were rational and unwavering, and that there were no familial pressures that pushed her to take this stance. When he was satisfied, he then considered the child's minor status, which strengthened the mother's right to determine the kind of therapies that could be offered her son. At the same time, the clinical data, together with the patient's youth, led the administrator to dismiss the possibility of court action. He then stated that he thought this was the right thing to do, from a moral stance. Finally, the medical student cited the child's clinical condition as the basis of decision-making and was then influenced by the strength of the mother's moral convictions. The possibility of legal liability was less salient to him than to his resident, who cited the clinical grounds for the rightness of the decision.

In essence I have suggested that the three perspectives consist of developmental changes that can be characterized as ranges. I then argued that these perspectives may coexist without competition as long as they serve the congruent interests of the patient, physician, and hospital administrator. Where there is conflict, each party ranks the competing perspectives on a principle of self-interest, with the medical, legal, and moral perspectives respectively assuming foremost importance to the medical student, the hospital administrator, and the patient. For each, the ranking of the two remaining perspectives remains open.

In this discussion of the three perspectives, much emphasis has been placed on identifying the absence of legal and moral perspectives in clinical practice. Furthermore, I have underscored how the perspectives differ. Significantly less discussion has been devoted to those situations where the perspectives converge, so that the treatment of choice is also the legally responsible thing to do and the morally correct course of action. It is by discerning absence and difference that one can begin to identify the implicit rules of professional decision-making within the medical context.

In the next three chapters on professional socialization, discussion will focus on how medical students acquire these perspectives. Medical students learn to abandon the role of the layperson and to order their perspectives in the fashion of physicians. This transition in perspectives is an important feature of socialization; it is tantamount to survival.

PART THREE

Socialization to Survival

8 The Second-year Student

With the first-year academic program behind them, second-year students have forgotten about how much they worried about getting into University Medical School; instead, they now congratulate themselves on having survived the first year, with its forty hours a week of scheduled lectures, plus all the additional hours spent in study. Admission to medical school gives students little reason to change their strategy for success. They continue to be as competitive, compulsive, and aggressive as they were as undergraduates. Over the next three years, students learn that one does not complete medical school; one survives it.

During the second year at University Medical School, students are given responsibility for patient care. This contributes to the ascendancy of a clinical perspective, which is reinforced by institutional constraints and role demands. Within the year students learn that survival is contingent on the adoption of the clinical perspective, with the legal and ethical perspectives subordinate to it. (The third and fourth years will be discussed in chapters 9 and 10.) The critical experience of the second year is the assumption of some clinical responsibility for patients. This contrasts with the first-year program, when for one academic semester students in groups of ten practice history-taking and physical examination under the aegis of a supervising physician. This clinical work is integrated into the basic science program with its emphasis on organ systems; however, according to the catalogue description, this supervised experience is to educate the student toward the goal of considering "the whole patient and his environment, rather than the disease process." To the second-year student, concern with "the whole patient" means concern with the psychological, social, and ethical aspects of each case as well as its clinical features. Later in his training, concern with "the whole patient" means concern with the totality of body organ systems.

This chapter will begin to suggest how the second-year student tries to fulfill the promise of the medical school catalogue, only to learn that many physicians at University Hospital are more concerned with the etiology of pathology in a given organ than in the psychosocial components of illness in a patient. While examples were given in chapter 7 of how an attending physician may direct the student's attention toward this broader view, the more frequent situation is one of disregard for the totality of illness as a human experience.

In keeping with the discussion of three perspectives (the clinical, the legal, and the moral), one can look at the second-year medical student with an interest in how he acquires or rejects these perspectives in the course of his initial clinical experience.[1] I shall argue that socialization to survival in the second year entails learning to think like a physician, with the concomitant emphasis on the clinical perspective. For most students the successful completion of the second year involves repudiating a highly personal and moralistic perspective, and substituting a professional perspective.

Students at University Hospital are assigned to two four-week rotations in medicine and one eight-week rotation in surgery (While lectures are scheduled for the second-year student in order to increase the amount of information at his disposal, they also serve the latent function of providing rest periods in which the student can consolidate energy for the next clinical rotation.) The medicine rotations are usually split between two locations, usually University Hospital and either Veterans', Community, or Center-City Hospital. Generally two second-year students are assigned to a medical service, which frequently has a third-year student doing a junior internship. The staff of each service consists of two interns, one resident, and one or more attending physicians. The rotation of members is staggered; house officers have usually been on a service a week before the arrival of second-year students. Attending physicians serve for four-week periods and arrive on a service the same week as students. Second-year students can be identified by their white jackets, their green name tags, and the frequent appearance of being lost or puzzled. When I informed some participating house officers that I would be studying how second-year students turn into physicians, the resident quipped, "Very slowly."

Until one is familiar with the schedule and pressures the second-year student encounters, it is difficult to understand why some concerns are emphasized at the expense of others. For example, why does the student learn it is more important to memorize the lab values for kidney electrolytes than to know the social history of the patient? The factors of sleep deprivation and lack of time for relaxation contribute to a standard of performance which is foreign to the typical layperson.

One of the key institutional constraints on the student's role performance is time. On paper, the second-year student's schedule looks like this:

A.M.

8:00–9:15	Work rounds	Monday–Saturday
9:15–11:00	Teaching rounds	Monday–Saturday (except Wednesday when there are grand rounds)
11:00–12:00	Time for scut	

P.M.

Noon–1:00	Teaching conference	Monday–Friday
1:00–2:00	Teaching fellow's conference	Monday, Wednesday, Friday
1:30–2:30	Radiology conference	Tuesday, Thursday
2:00–3:00	Dermatology conference	Wednesday

This day extends on both ends, with hours spent on reading, taking histories, doing physical examinations, writing up work-ups, preparing presentations for teaching rounds, and doing scut. Scut consists of routine laboratory work, such as drawing blood samples, making slides, calling labs for test results, reviewing x-rays, and ordering consultations. Because of this schedule, lack of sleep is a daily complaint. The student who complains of having had only three hours' sleep is likely to be answered by the intern completing his chartwork from the night before, "Well, that's three hours more than I had." During one day, with one admission assigned to him, Tom Watts, a second-year student, did not start his work-up till 8 P.M. He spent two hours on the history-taking and physical examination, an hour or more on the scut, and several hours on the write-up and preparation for the presentation. Before 8 A.M. the next morning he had to check on his patients, pick up x-rays and lab data, and try to grab some breakfast. His intern's favorite piece of advice was "move like the wind." The importance of using time wisely reminds us that neither overly scheduled people nor exhausted people have the time to reflect on ethics.

Since the second-year student is at a loss to know how to do anything except as described in *Harrison's Principles of Internal Medicine*, he is eager for pieces of advice, "pearls," which will contribute to both speed and competence. Efficiency alleviates some of the psychological stress of fulfilling expectations of competence. While *Principles of Internal Medicine* is the Bible of the medical student and a resource throughout his medical career, it is primarily a sourcebook for the etiology of disease, pathology, diagnosis, prognosis, and management. It does not provide "how to" information, such as how to do an electrocardiogram, nor does it guide the student in the recognition of the atypical or nonclassical case. Consequently, the second-year student has to seek out willing teachers to instruct him in standard operations, such as how to use a "butterfly" syringe.

A second kind of advice consists of "tricks." Tricks are skillful ways of doing something, often short cuts or special techniques that facilitate a difficult procedure. The teaching resident announced that "there is a trick to examining axilla [armpits]." The second-year student boasts, "Samson showed me this trick last night."

Sometimes more advanced students or house officers volunteer advice, based on self-identification: "When I was a student someone had to tell me. . . ." Sometimes the student makes a direct request for information or demonstration of a technique. Occasionally the student interprets unsolicited advice as unnecessary and is likely to feel debased by the assumption of his ignorance.

Finally, advice can be offered negatively as well as positively, though the latter is more common. Positive advice takes the form of, "Always record the lab data someplace on the chart because people tend to stuff the lab slips in their pockets, and they are never charted." Negative advice is often given to restrain the student's enthusiasm for certain procedures: "The important thing is to remember not to go biopsing all these people with. . . . Wait a month before deciding." Thus, "pearls" alleviate anxiety by emphasizing the clinical perspective. "Pearls" concerning ethics are rare or nonexistent.

Early in his clinical experience the medical student becomes a student of probability, as the use of percentages and betting terms demonstrates. Once again, this assuages anxiety arising from uncertainty. The listing of possible diagnoses in descending order of probability is a common way of structuring the differential diagnosis:

> For example, a patient comes in and complains of loss of weight. The student must determine the magnitude of the loss. He then must find out whether the loss of weight reflects normal (or increased appetite) or decreased appetite. If the former, it may signify hyperthyroidism, intestinal cancer, or diabetes. If the latter, it may indicate psychological causes, gastro-intestinal problems, or systemic disturbances. If systemic disturbances are indicated, the student must look for: (1) malignancy, (2) infection, (3) uremia (kidney failure), (4) cardio-vascular disease, (5) endocrine-metabolic disorders, (6) intoxication from lead or alcohol, and (7) hematologic [blood] disorders. After listing all the possible causes of the admitting complaint, the student must enumerate what procedures must be done in order to rule out each of the possibilities.[2]

When a student reviews the differential diagnosis with the attending physician, he is expected to understand the etiology of the disease. In subsequent years the student will be held responsible for diagnosis and management (including medication). But the prime emphasis of the second year is on understanding how pathology comes to exist, with the rationale that conceptual knowledge outlasts changes in diagnosis and management. Despite acknowledgment of the exotica in academic medicine—"Cadillac medicine," as the house officers call it—the bias remains in favor of the common, or statistically probable diagnosis.* A common aphorism is, "If you hear the sound of horses' hoofs, don't go looking for zebras." When the medical student does find a true "zebra," it is a source of great delight. It allows him to bask in his medical acumen. It is the crowning touch to an "interesting" case. Furthermore, it is a claim to status which is not bounded by "what a second-year student should know." It is a respectable performance for any physician.

When a student knows something that might not be expected of him, he may offer an explanation based on luck: "I just happened to be reading about this diagnosis," or "I saw this on my last rotation." There is always latent pride in these manifest statements of humility,

---

*Cadillac medicine is medicine for the few by the few, or the use of highly specialized physicians to treat clinical exotica. It was not uncommon for grand rounds to discuss a rare hemoglobin disorder found on the west coast of Africa.

and the tension between the two comes out when one student asks another, "Did you know that before you got this patient?" The idea that one's peers may already know the diagnostic signs of, say, cerebellar ataxia, when one's own experience provides no basis for such clinical expertise, creates discomfort. It leads to assumptions that one is not studying or retaining as much as one's peers, and is thus a reflection of personal inadequacy. Alternatively, one may feel that one's assumption of "what a second-year student should know" is incorrect. Consequently, the second-year student is vulnerable to fears of failure. The way to alleviate these fears is to subscribe to the clinical perspective.

One way of gaining control over the situation of uncertainty is to see matters in clearly demarcated blacks and whites. The student divides knowledge into two spheres: what he knows, and what he does not know but ought to. In the case of the teaching conference the student knows that all the students in attendance have not had identical clinical courses; consequently he can excuse his ignorance by saying that the respondent must have learned the information in a course he has not had. Eventually the student will begin to realize that even the best of physicians do not have all the answers, and many things are unknown within medicine. But at this early stage of socialization, situations which require statements of judgment and an individualized approach are exceedingly anxiety-provoking. The student is more secure when he knows exactly what is known and where to find it.

The institutional constraint of an extremely hierarchical organization reinforces the tension between role ideal and role performance. Social stratification within the hospital bureaucracy aggravates the student's psychological discomfort. Everywhere the student looks he sees people who seem to have more knowledge and more confidence than he. Their survival is ensured, while his is in doubt. It sometimes occurs to him that the ancillary members of the team—the nurses, the practical nurses, the aides, the respiratory therapist— appear to know more than a second-year student. This conflicts with what he knows to be the truth: they will be lifelong subordinates to him within the hierarchy. Medical students, no matter what their degree of clinical incompetence, subscribe to the notion that a fledgling physician is superior to any nonphysician member of the health-care team. The need to accept the helpful corrections of the nurses aggravates the student's insecurity and makes him resentful of the nurses' casual ease and confidence.

The most common and most effective setting for the socialization of medical students is the nearly daily teaching rounds. Teaching rounds free the student from the delusion that the recommendations of the house officers are based on personal eccentricity. More important, they provide opportunities for refining skills of differential diagnosis and patient management. The second-year student has difficulty in appreciating the latter facet of rounds, because he is still caught up in the recognition of disease. Additional functions of teaching rounds include (1) the documentation of the scope and nature of medical knowledge, including the particular form of thinking that is part of professional performance;[3] (2) the identification of the limits of both professional and individual capabilities; (3) the need for cooperative efforts across institutional boundaries, both internal and external to University Hospital; and (4) the establishment of a principle of public performance based on the visibility of mistakes to colleagues and superiors through written records and oral presentations. This extends to the "mortality board" which reviews the cases of all patients who die on hospital services.

An important part of teaching rounds is the presentation of cases to the attending physician. In any good presentation there is a claim to knowledge based on history-taking and physical examination which purports to yield a statement of universality and reliability, such that anyone performing the same operations would make the identical observations and comparable recommendations for management and prognosis. A good presentation is brief and well organized, and includes all relevant clinical material. It is constructed to demonstrate conceptual understanding as well as rote recall of laboratory data. It avoids "wastebasket" terms of no significant reliability, such as *pseudolymphoma*.*

The second-year student struggles to make a good presentation as a condition of his interaction with the attending physician. If, after his performance, the student's intern believes he was too slow or too verbose or insufficiently clear about the clinical facts of the case, he

---

Pseudolymphoma is used to describe the growth of abnormal tissue which resembles malignancies, and for which there is no apparent explanation.

will deny the student the privilege of "taking up the attending physician's time." He will tell the student that he needs more practice and can get that practice by presenting to the intern or the resident. In the course of quizzing the student and offering a critique of his performance, the attending physician will impress upon the student the need for growth, in terms of developing clinical judgment and contributing to the corpus of medical knowledge. When the attending physician asks, "Now suppose you are the resident and a patient presents with . . . , What will you do?" he expects the student to have a succinct and competent answer, based on the clinical facts of the case. This is the fundamental goal of "presenting" and the related quizzing, and this focus contributes to the absence of moral or legal discussion.

Quizzing goes on between the attending physician and the student, between the house officer and the student, and sometimes between student and student. The following is an example of quizzing, which is typical because it stresses the clinical questions. It is an example of latent socialization because it teaches the student that the clinical perspective is the important one.

Attending physician: How many blood cultures did you collect?

Student: Three.

Attending physician: That's the standard number. Do you do blood cultures in this case?

Student. Yes.

Attending physician: No, they won't grow.

Student: I've run down to the lab with blood cultures here.

Attending physician: Did they grow?

Student: No, but not much that I sent down did grow.

Attending physician: Did you get a urinalysis?

Student: Sounds reasonable.

Attending physician: But is it?

Quizzing forces the student to "focus in" on the significant findings of the case, to enumerate the so-called problems, to propose a differential diagnosis, and to consider the possible plan of management. When it is followed up with review of the associated physical findings, as is the case with teaching rounds, the student has the opportunity to compare the scope and depth of his synthesis with that of the attending physician. The attending physician walks into the patient's room with his entourage, introduces himself and the team, and highlights the relevant points of the physical exam. He asks the patient a few questions, and then withdraws from the room with the team. In the hall or the conference room he discusses the patient, asks further questions, answers questions, and then listens to the next presentation before repeating the routine. In this way the student learns to set goals, to evaluate performance, and to grow comfortable with some variation in diagnostic techniques and work styles. This gives the student some way of measuring weakness and growth on an almost daily basis.

The second-year student rehearses for hours before his presentation to the attending physician and the ensuing quizzing. The student may display fear in pressured speech or an unnatural tonality of voice, though this tends to decrease quickly after the first few times. Clearly the ability to withstand the test of quizzing enhances self-esteem. Conversely, a bad performance can be devastating. All the attending physician need say is, "You'd better get to work," and the student becomes a mass of nerves till he makes a successful presentation.

Aside from the student's need to test his own limits, and as a way of evaluating his fulfillment of role demands, the student also learns that professional behavior is affected by interaction with other physicians: local physicians, private admitting physicians, and consulting physicians. He becomes aware of the existence of hospital support services and their personnel: social workers, dietitians, physical therapists. When there are low levels of trust with respect to any of these people or services, a "crisis of confidence" develops. This often entails an insidious hierarchy of medical services, with comparisons between different kinds of specialists, different kinds of professional training, or the relative skills of the local physician versus the University Hospital house staff.[4] These comparisons impinge on the definition of "appropriate therapy." The second-year student must learn to decode the preferences of the house staff with regard to these variables in order to understand why he is given contradictory or seemingly nonrational instructions when he asks, "What shall I do?"

Student: I think this patient has cellulitis. The intern says it may be a septic joint, so I should call rheumatology. It took forty-five minutes to get through to the person on call. I had the resident look at it. He says it may be osteo, so I should get a film. I've never seen it, so I ask him, "Do you really think so?" He says, "No, but get a film." So I'm getting a film.

The failure to use resources is common in University Hospital. In part this grows out of unwillingness to delegate responsibility for fear that it may contribute to undermining authority. The delegation of responsibility also necessitates the positive evaluation of subordinates in the hierarchy. This physicians implicitly refuse to do, because it suggests that they can be replaced by those who are subordinate to them by virtue of less formal education and different kinds of clinical experience. Physicians tend to refer their patients to people of inferior status only when they define the situation as hopeless or after other avenues of lateral and upward referral have been exhausted. Thus, patients are referred to psychiatrists only when there is no explanatory organic pathology and where the healing power of the patient-physician relationship fails to yield improvement. The more common tack is to discharge the patient, knowing that the patient will continue to shop around for a physician (or quack) who will do what the patient wants.

Thus, the second-year student learns about the "neurons," the "pulmos," and "the renal men"—the neurologists, the pulmonary specialists, and the kidney specialists—who are requested to evaluate patients on the medical service and to offer their opinion. The recommendations of consulting physicians ("consults") are not binding, though they often clarify an ambiguous situation. When contradictory opinions are offered, as is frequently the case, it falls to the resident in consultation with the attending physician and the responsible intern or third-year student to decide on a course of action. The ultimate decision belongs to the resident.

The second-year student often resists the suggestion that he, rather than the intern, initiate the consult request, because of the intimidating prospect of having to talk to a person of established competence who frequently has a reputation as "a noted authority." The student fears that technical discussion will go past him. Some consultation services achieve notoriety because of their dislike for teaching or because they constantly play "hard to reach" in order to avoid additional duties. A specialty like neurology may be characterized as attracting physicians who use very technical language to give the impression that they are exceptionally competent. The student may try to minimize contact with such a consult and lose the opportunity to force the neurologist into clarifying the situation for him. When the house officer meets up with student resistance to a consult, he is likely to push, saying, "You'll learn something, and it may help the patient."

The second-year student must learn to distinguish between personal and collective evaluations of behavior. He may try to resist the subtle pressure to internalize these biases as a means to identification with a specific professional circle, such as physicians in "medicine" (as opposed to surgery). Examples of such bias include the following:

Attending physician: My inclination is that you guys are probably smarter than they are, knowing Garden City Hospital. I would repeat the GI series.

Attending physician: I can forgive you for accepting the data, but anyone who knows those butchers [surgeons] should know they don't know anything about electrolytes.

Resident: Has urology seen her? Not if I can help it. They would be pulling a stone out every ten minutes.

Consulting physician: Psychiatrists think that just by talking to one of their patients, you endanger their psychological condition.

The basis of role identity is in the group. From very early in his medical career the student learns that professional identity is founded in collective activity. He is quickly introduced to the importance of professional etiquette. While one may be openly chastised by any of the house officers, the attending physician, or even the nurses, one's superiors should never be directly confronted with their inferior level of performance. Even when there is valid reason to believe the private physician incompetent, one learns to circumvent the limits of the relationship, by suggesting the need for a consult, or by doing the relevant tests as well as the irrelevant ones the private physician has requested. Within the social relations of the team, the attending physician will never openly criticize the performance of the resident, and rarely that of the interns. Informally, strong suggestions for changes in behavior may be broached, quite frequently in the form of the collective "we": "We physicians sometimes have difficulty in ridding ourselves of obsolescent techniques."

The recurrent criticism of the local physician reflects this concern with group standards of performance. In university circles the local physician is a negative role model. It is repeatedly argued that the independent practitioner lacks the stimulation of his peers, which is a necessary incentive for keeping up with the literature and refining skills. "Local doc" (LMD) is a term of opprobrium. If the student should imply that he desires to become a general practitioner, he is strongly advised, "One can't do everything and expect to be good at anything." Even the possibility of being board-certified in both medicine and pediatrics is suspect, for the same reason. The boundaries of acceptable behavior are narrowly defined for the second-year student, and without the knowledge or experience to challenge them, he accepts them like any other condition of survival.

It has been suggested that the second-year student learns the norms of his role through structured interaction with supervising house staff. The set of role models is expanded by the use of consulting physicians and the student's introduction to a succession of advisors, research supervisors, and academic professors in the course of his career. This is in contrast to nurses, social workers, and other allied medical workers who are rejected as role models, even when some of their traits might aid the medical student's survival. The student tends to reject them as models because they are not trained as physicians, and therefore are assumed to be less intelligent, less trained, and subordinate to the student. In reality they may be more experienced, more intelligent, and more mature, though cast in an institutionally subordinate position. Nurses, for example, learn to anticipate the arrogance of the medical student and to manipulate his inadequacy by withholding helpful information until the student is about "to go under," at which time they sweetly suggest that next time he might try what has worked for them. The student slinks away grateful for the rescue.

Students also learn from their experiences with patients what is expected of them, which contributes to their idealized notions of professional behavior. They learn that patients expect their caretakers to introduce themselves as "doctor," to proceed with confidence and a gentle touch, and to comport themselves with evidence of dedication to the profession. Since patients implicitly identify physicians with a clinical perspective, they tend to pull the second-year student toward it by their use of praise to reward him for "acting like a good little doctor." When second-year students walk into the room and announce their student status and see the patient blanch, they learn they have violated patient expectations. They learn to award themselves an honorific "doctor" and to summon enough self-confidence to act like physicians.

When students no longer fear for their daily survival, they can begin to take their own psychological needs into account. After the initial thrill of having patients, second-year students must come to terms with their predilection for some kinds of patients and their distaste for others.[5] There evolves a definition of the "good patient," just as there is a definition of the "good physician." For the second-year student the "good patient" is one who has a clear history, who has no real complications in the physical findings, and who does not require "a lot of complicated management stuff."

The second-year student also develops a preference for acutely ill patients over the chronically ill. He finds patients with psychological problems the least desirable. The acutely ill patient is desirable because there is a great amount of satisfaction in seeing a patient get better. This is analogous to the surgeon's claim of the superiority of surgery to medicine. While nobody wants a patient who is so sick that there are overwhelming odds of mortality, the physician-in-training learns to appreciate how good management can yield dramatic results. Chronic patients are less favored because they tend to have multiple medical problems which require a large investment of time with a moderate payoff. Second-year students find almost any medical problem exciting in the initial encounter, but novelty soon fades into routine.

As much as the second-year student aspires to treat all of his patients alike, the realities of the clinical milieu make it a near impossibility. The second-year student must learn to confront his preferences, compensate where possible, and formulate some way of minimizing the "unwanted" patient in subsequent career choices. The medical student who hates dealing with elderly patients and their long problem lists will avoid such specialties as geriatrics, oncology, and probably cardiology. He may plan to specialize in pediatrics, where the child frequently presents with an acute illness and then gets better quickly. In the interim the student will choose electives from services which attract their patients from younger sectors of the population: obstetrics, dermatology, and psychiatry.

The overwhelming fear of the second-year student is that he will botch the patient's chances for recovery by acts of commission or omission, through inadequate technique or inappropriate discourse. Students learn that they should not tell the patient too much in order to avoid self-fulfilling prophecies and additional work for themselves. A self-fulfilling prophecy occurs when the social actor's confidence "in erroneous information generates its own spurious confirmation."[6] It is regularly demonstrated that patients learn after repeated questioning from their many examiners what physicians are looking for; they begin to model their responses after the suggested symptoms. Of course, "If a patient walks like a duck and sounds like a duck, what do you assume?" The supposition that the patient may be a genuine "duck" requires a work-up to rule out that possibility. The second-year student, like any other student, does not wish to create unnecessary work for himself.

As the second-year student grows more secure, he wishes to expand the boundaries of his capabilities; yet the student must consider whether he is exposing the patient to significant risk. Each time the student considers suggesting an alternative to the recommended treatment as proposed by his intern or attending physician, he weighs the possibility of an incriminating admission of incompetence. When the probability of mistakes is greater than that of appropriate recommendations, it is difficult for the student to assume he is correct in his doubts. Therefore, as a technique of survival, he considers all the angles before venturing an opinion that contradicts a superior.

Part of the reason the second-year student lacks the courage of his convictions is that he still addresses problems from the perspective of a layperson, while he knows he should be thinking like a physician. As the student develops greater clinical acumen and learns to arm himself with citations from the literature, he becomes bolder in his challenges. But the second-year student has frail clinical resources, and he is fearful of invoking "personal" reasoning. Without even four years of clinical experience, one can hardly expect to evoke consideration by saying, "In my personal experience. . . ."

When a second-year student suggested that a patient had the right to know he had cancer, the attending physician suggested it might be sufficient to inform the patient that he had "a serious tumor." He cautioned the student that "in my experience" patients rarely want the truth. He advised that when they want to know, they will ask. When the student was still unsatisfied, the attending physician recommended that the student sit down with his patient and evaluate whether he already understood his diagnosis. The attending physician was addressing a question of ethics obliquely by the citation of his clinical experience. This technique is frequently used to manage ethical issues through the convergence of perspectives. The student debated what he should do and decided he would speak with the patient, for if he were in the patient's place, he would want to know. After talking with the patient at length, he realized that the patient did not want to know the gravity of his illness and had not assimilated the information about his tumor.

Second-year students have difficulty restricting themselves to the clinical perspective, though they gradually learn that survival entails incorporating "detachment" into a positive self-image. The second-year student's confrontation with death illustrates the problem of thinking like a physician when one also wishes to acknowledge the humanity of the patient. Second-year students tended to use me as "mother-confessor," since I was not identified with their teachers, and because they were pleased to find someone who would listen to their problems. Therefore, they would come to me with their reports of how badly they felt when their first patients "went down the tubes."*

A patient died of iatrogenic causes (the negative consequences of treatment). He had come to the hospital for routine prostate surgery, suffered from critical postsurgical complications which included infection in the chest cavity, and then bled to death when an artery was nicked during a surgical procedure to drain the chest cavity of excess fluids and pus. George Atkins confessed, "It followed me home all weekend. There we were, Alan [another second-year student] and me, holding each other, wondering why it happened." There was still an element of disbelief in his narrative, even though two days had passed. When I asked him whether anything might have prepared him for what he saw and felt, he answered, "I hope not. I do not want to lose my sensitivity to death and my patients. I want to feel comfortable with dying patients. I want to be able to help them die." The resident, on

---

*In hospital lingo "to go down the tubes" is to die; the etymology is unclear. It is an objectifying term which equates death with disappearance. Frequently the deceased patient does seem to disappear, once the post-mortem care is complete. It can be difficult to spot when the orderly has arrived with the litter as well as when he leaves, because once death has occurred, attention is immediately directed to the viable patients. See David Sudnow, *Passing On* (Englewood Cliffs, N.J.: Prentice-Hall, 1960).

the other hand, was quoted as saying, "I won't let anyone else be tapped like that."

When second-year students seek information about how and when a patient has died, they receive only the briefest answer: "At seven this morning," or "We closed the curtains, and he was dead when we opened them." While the students are not openly chastised for asking, the message is clear: medical attention should be directed to the living. In time the second-year students become more astute in presenting their questions, and eventually they cease asking them.

Similarly, second-year students maintain some sensitivity to the nonmedical components of illness, though it is generally minimized as they continue their clinical education, for reasons which will be elaborated later.[7]

Second-year student: My patient is depressed and says things like "what I need is a new body."

Resident: When you're breathless, you can't breathe, and you feel like you are dying all the time.

Student: He seems depressed. What are the psychological aspects of pneumonia patients?

Resident: It may be more difficult to be a pneumo cripple than a renal cripple, because we are more conscious of the former's function than the latter.

Attending physician: Does he have children? Maybe you can change the focus from him to them. If he can keep his children from smoking, then he's done something positive. But the fact is, he's a pulmonary cripple.

The resident acknowledges the possibility of depression, but treats it in clinical terms; the attending physician provides something for the student to do for the patient. Neither suggests a psychiatric consult, or a social service consultation, or reevaluating the patient's inhalation therapy with the respiration therapist, or letting the patient talk with another pulmonary patient who has come to terms with his impairment. The student has not benefited from any instruction on the psychiatric evaluation of a depressed patient. There is a subtle message of irritation with the student's concern with this "problem," which encourages the student to drop the question. Students try to maintain cordial relations with physicians because they fear they will become objects of the physicians' irritation; the irritated attending physician will be a more critical and more demanding instructor than one who is not annoyed. Therefore, the student learns to avoid irritating the attending physician by asking "unwanted" questions.

It may well be that part of the attending physician's irritation reflects his own difficulty in handling these problems directly. Even house staff who demonstrate concern with "ethical issues" express some difficulty in joining their clinical and ethical concerns. Yet while the honest expression of confusion might strengthen the attractiveness of role models, house staff tend to take less direct routes in managing their own role confusion.

Also, while role models do exist who support an ethical perspective in conjunction with the clinical and legal perspectives, they have little perceptible effect on students. Perhaps at a later time, with fewer pressing demands and in higher positions in the hierarchy, students will draw on them as role models.

However, students who are constantly fatigued and under great pressure to perform, who are regularly confronted with the need to adjust to new services and new co-workers, and who question the appropriateness of their calling, are ready subjects for the adoption of group norms, as the literature on social movements and "brainwashing" suggest.[8] For at least six years the student's energies and attention have been directed at becoming a physician. Since entering medical school, the student has lived medicine. In the words of the theme song of the 1975 "Freshman Follies":

> I haven't had fun
> Since the damn thing's begun,
> I haven't been laid,
> I'm intellectually frayed,
> I'm losing the charm I once had.

With the completion of the second year of University Medical School, the student concludes that he has survived the worst of the medical student experience. The bulk of classroom work is over, with only one or two academic electives remaining. The initial fears of failure have been moderated by seeing patients get better under one's care. Informally the student may express the belief that somehow he is now a "different" person, though the basis of this change is often unclear to him. But there is the underlying awareness that in the course of these months on clinical services one has become more of a physician and less of a layperson. This is symbolically illustrated by the student's frequent use of the honorific "doctor" when he calls up outside physicians or the laboratory services.

While one may have expected that the second-year student would be initiated into "medical ethics," especially considering his malleability and concern with "the whole patient," experience reveals the contrary. The major ethical issue of the second-year student is "truth-telling": How much does the patient have a right to know? Three examples have been given: confronting the death of a patient from iatrogenic causes, coping with a depressed patient with a chronic disease, and dealing with a patient who denies the seriousness of his illness. A fourth kind of case is the patient who is under experimental protocol through tacit consent.

> Mrs. Laurie Jansen, a thirty-eight-year-old mother of three children, the eldest being twelve years old, had spent the better part of the last six months coming in and out of the hospital for treatment of end-stage Hodgkin's disease, a form of cancer. One by one the conventional means of treating her disease were exhausted, and she was put under a protocol for use of an experimental "poison," a very potent three-drug combination therapy. When the second-year student asked the attending physician whether Mrs. Jansen knew about the protocol and about the risks of her therapy, the physician merely replied, "She knows we are trying to offer her a viable option. We have her confidence." There was no further discussion as the troupe of students and house staff moved on to the next patient.

The student is rewarded for a lack of concern with ethical issues through institutional constraints on his behavior as well as role-related and psychological factors. Institutional constraints include such contingencies as (1) time, (2) the status hierarchy, (3) referrals, with their own rules of direction and rank ordering, (4) interaction with patients, and (5) role models whose demonstrated concern is with "viable" patients. These factors tend to force the student into an emphasis on the clinical perspective.

This bias in favor of the clinical perspective is aided by role demands which emphasize (1) efficiency, (2) solicitation of advice from superiors, (3) meritorious performance on teaching rounds, (4) interaction with other physicians (consultants, local physicians, and private attending physicians), and (5) a collective orientation toward "medical" services (as opposed to surgical services).

In addition, there are psychological factors which work toward alleviating a sense of inadequacy and inexperience on the part of the second-year student. Uncertainty (of diagnosis, procedural competence, performance, and so on) and status anxiety cause the student to seek solutions in "cut-and-dry" thought processes, as in the manipulation of probabilities and the rigid calculation of "what I know" versus "what I do not know." The student's fears and anxieties are abetted by the appearance of subordinates who seem to know more than he does, as well as the need to make "good" presentations to the attending physician almost daily. Furthermore, the student worries whether he will get "good" patients, or whether he will be saddled with "difficult" patients or, worse, "turkeys."

Consequently, the first year of significant clinical responsibility is also the year of gradual extinction of the ethical perspective, because of its identification with the personal perspective of the layperson. The legal perspective has little meaning for the second-year student and thus does not intrude on his consciousness. But the clinical perspective is held out as the mainstay of his professional identity. The student actively works to internalize the behavior, vocabulary, and manner of thinking of the physician.

9 The Third-year Student

The third-year student believes the worst is behind him as he prepares for his internship through the rite of passage known as the junior internship. There is no medical student so compulsive as the junior intern in pursuit of an "honors" grade and an enthusiastic recommendation for an internship. He knows the next four weeks will be difficult, but he also knows that the satisfactory completion of this rotation will attest to his ability to perform satisfactorily as an intern. While one may question this equation of competence, since one four-week rotation hardly equals the fifty-two weeks of an internship, the discrepancy never seems to worry the third-year student. It is a symbolic event, signifying his capacity to survive the rigors of the practice of medicine.

In examining the socialization of the third-year student, I shall note two broad changes, the second subordinate to the first: (1) the acceptance of the clinical perspective as the pervasive modality of thinking, for it becomes second nature to the third-year student; and (2) the acquisition of self-confidence which allows critical thinking. I shall also argue that the ethical perspective becomes something of an afterthought for the third-year student. He is reflective *after* the rotation, not during it. This contributes to the conservation of energy, and the third-year student is continually struggling to be "on top of his patients."

Once again, the reasons for these changes are founded in institutional constraints, role demands, and psychological factors. Institutional constraints consist of the pressure of time and the social stratification within the hospital system. The student is closely supervised by the resident while he gradually expands his responsibility for

patients. The student hopes that there will be enough patients to provide a variety of diagnoses, but not so many that the house staff finds it
easier and more efficient to work up patients themselves. As the student acquires more responsibility, his self-confidence increases, psy-
chologically reinforcing his allegiance to the clinical perspective.

The junior intern is required to do all his own admissions,
though they are subject to the review of the resident. The junior intern
is "up" for admissions every other day and on call every third night.
The night call usually consists of admitting patients from 3 P.M. to 8
A.M., though there is some variation across services. The junior intern
is responsible for the daily scut of his patients, the continual planning
of the management of their problems, the writing of doctor's orders,
including medications, testing, and diet, and the charting of lab data
and progress notes. Everything that becomes part of the written record
is co-signed by either the resident or one of the interns.

The junior intern is constantly under fire, and he must develop
coping mechanisms, which include a thick skin, a sense of humor, the
ability to go without sleep, and fleetness of foot as he runs up and
down the stairs to the labs and x-ray department because the elevators
are too slow and he is too impatient to wait for the data to arrive by
messenger. He has the comfort of knowing "this too shall pass," and
for a month he can put up with almost anything. While these defenses
protect him, they are not conducive to involvement with patients as
people. In the course of a typical day, excluding time spent with a
patient during an admissions work-up, the student will spend less than
fifteen minutes with each of his two to seven patients. He will spend
most of his time doing scut, which reaches gigantic proportions with
"a really sick patient."* In such instances he will have to draw blood
and do blood gases several times a day, calibrate respirators and other
technological support systems, and repeatedly evaluate lab data for
needed changes in management.

Since the third-year student doing a junior internship has no
scheduled lectures, he may devote all his hours to medicine, which
frequently means days, nights, and weekends. The remarks about

---

*"A really sick patient" is acutely ill and requires legitimate medical attention,
as contrasted with "a sick patient," who requires neither intensive nursing nor the
comprehensive attention of the physician. The "turkey" is defined as "not really
sick."

sleeplessness continue, but now they originate in being on call for upwards of sixty hours straight over weekends.

The third-year student starts out fearing the new responsibilities. He is slow and methodical in his work-ups. Before preparing prescriptions for the house officer's signature he has to consult both the resident and the hospital formulary (the publication which lists medications and supplies stocked in the hospital pharmacy along with recommended dosages and listings of equivalent drugs). On the one hand, he fears that he is not giving enough of himself to his patients; on the other, he worries that he cannot absorb their demands for his time and still get everything done. He wonders how many diagnostic procedures are necessary before he can establish a diagnosis with confidence. Occasionally he worries about the financial cost to the patient. When he gets "a really sick patient," he worries that the patient will "go down the tubes" because of something he does or does not do, but soon he is so involved in writing orders for his patient that he cannot afford the time to worry. He collects massive amounts of data and hopes he will not have to explain the significance of the information before he has figured it out. When he can report that he is "on top of all his patients" he is buoyant with his own accomplishments:

Third-year student: I feel good today because I am on top of all my patients. I want to be on top of all my patients all the time, knowing everything there is to know about their cases. Then I'll be happy.

When he is buried under all the work left to be done in a day, the student is tenacious in refusing the resident's offer of assistance "if it is too much for you."

As the weeks progress, he becomes increasingly like an intern. He wants a "beeper" so he can be paged in the cafeteria. When he does have occasion to carry one, he is thrilled to be pulled away from friends who are beeper-less. Another way in which he acts like an intern is in his willingness to offer a second-year student a "pearl," or his availability to assist in drawing blood from "a bad vein."

The use of probabilities is an established tool of problem-solving for the third-year student. He has some crude sense of which is a more probable diagnosis. As the student becomes more familiar with the literature, he enjoys the control acquired by being able to cite statistics: "Patients treated with medication *a* do better than patients treated with *b* 65 percent of the time." Students often made jokes about guessing the right diagnosis, and egged me into joining the betting: "Guess the right diagnosis and win a kewpie doll!" When they go against the odds and find "a zebra," they are momentarily "king of the mountain."

For example, David Hanson did a history and physical examination on Bertha Jackson, an obese black woman of fifty-eight who was admitted with a complaint of weight loss. The resident sent David off with the admonition, "You know and I know she has nothing wrong with her." As it turned out, David discovered that Bertha Johnson had undetected diabetes mellitus, despite the fact that she was under a physician's supervision for hypertension. The diagnosis had been overlooked by a physician who probably never tested her urine for sugar with a Dipstix, a ten-second test using a chemically impregnated slip of paper. Further exploration of her case revealed she had one nonfunctioning kidney, which made her "one very sick lady."

Because the third-year student is going beyond the boundaries of the textbook, he no longer holds to the simplistic model of black or white, right or wrong. The third-year student notes the component of the irrational in medicine and denigrates as naive anyone who subscribes to the principle that medicine is "a science." The student hears the house officers complain about the surgeon's use of prophylactic antibiotics, which one attending physician explained by saying, "Well, every man needs his superstition."[1] Furthermore, he sees that physicians have their favorite theories, which appear to work, even if there is no rational reason for their efficacy.

> Mrs. Arthur Jones complained of bizarre blackout spells and pains shooting down her neck and shoulder. After a complete physical, including exhaustive diagnostic tests, no organic basis for her complaint could be found.
>
> When Dr. Harvey White, her private physician and member of the house staff, was asked whether he wanted a psychiatrist consult, he replied, "She's getting better, so her problems must be getting better." The patient was never referred to the psychiatric service, and she did get better and return home.

Like the fraternity pledge, the third-year student is subject to the capriciousness of his fraternity brothers, who may test him for their own amusement and pleasure. In the emergency room one morning, a third-year student from another medical school (and thus an "outsider" from an "inferior" school) approached the intern and said, "I have this lady in room 9 with Crohn's disease." The intern immediately pounced on him. "How do you know it's Crohn's disease? How was the diagnosis made? Maybe Dr. Barker is wrong."* And then he apologized, "I am just giving you shit."

If the third-year student has some intrinsic self-confidence, he will learn to appreciate the suggestions of the nurses. If he is unsure of himself, he will resent their interference, and he will summarily dismiss them as shrews and bitches. They will let few opportunities go by to correct him, because they think he should learn to do things the right way. Sometimes they merely want to remedy his ignorance without making a point of it: "Why don't you try one of those orange needles? That's what most of the doctors like to use." On bad days, however, it seems like everyone is after him.

The overall fit between team members is a function of chance and professional standards of collegiality. Every student and physician can tell of that one horrendous rotation when student (or attending physician) and house officer were genuine enemies; but there is also the need to repress animosity in order to serve the patient's interests and the house staff's equanimity. Nevertheless, patients sometimes find themselves in the middle of house feuds. An additional source of irritation and dissatisfaction is the presence of less intelligent house officers than the University Hospital administrators would like to acknowledge as their own. While students will try to avoid these people, they do not always succeed, despite the practice of artful scheduling. When a student requests his rotations for the term, he gives ranked choices. He calculates general popularity, the availability of positions, fluctuations in demand based on the calendar, and class priorities. Students try to seek out residents and interns with whom they or friends have worked with satisfaction. They sometimes return to work with an intern who has advanced to his residency by the time of the student's junior internship.

Teaching rounds are less traumatic for the third-year student because he has mastered the form of the presentation and has some reasonable idea of what he must know to satisfy the attending physi-

---

*Dr. Barker was "a real honcho," the author of an important text in gastroenterology and respected throughout the medical community.

cian. The student has internalized the clinical perspective, with its objectification of the patient, and he no longer confronts the difficulty of incorporating ethical concerns into his presentation.

Third-year students get quizzed, though they may be less frequent targets if second-year students are on the same service; however, the quizzing of the third-year student is less of an implied challenge to the student's competence than it was the preceding year. The attending physician will focus on a single aspect of the presentation rather than testing the overall boundaries of the student's knowledge.

Part of the third-year student's instruction in professional etiquette stresses dealing with the "local docs," the LMD. Professional etiquette is a narrowly defined subset of "medical ethics" and more openly recognized than the kinds of ethical issues surrounding "truth-telling," control of reproduction, or "the right to die." Thus, the student is instructed on how to direct the LMD toward doing what the University Hospital physician thinks should be done without antagonizing the LMD:

Resident: You don't call up John Doe, M.D., and say, "Why the hell didn't you test for strep?" You merely suggest: "Don't you think we ought to do. . . . " Even if the guy doesn't know what you're talking about, he'll go along with your plan.

The bias against certain medical specialties becomes more established in the third-year student, especially once he realizes the existence of "the surgical personality" versus "the medicine man." While there are always enough students who "see the light" and dedicate themselves to becoming surgeons, those who are not so charmed by the tasks of stitching and cutting decide to stay in medicine. I was told the following joke by a third-year student:

Dr. McAlister, a famous surgeon, is getting into the elevator with his entourage. The last student in the group is slow in getting on and sticks his arm in the elevator door to force it open. Dr. McAlister scolds the guy, saying, "Save your hands. Someday you may want to be a surgeon. Use your head."

Surgeons are characterized as being less intelligent than people who go into "medicine." They are "anal types," arrogant, and inclined to "crack open a belly" rather than to try the slower route of pharmacological management. The third-year student tells how the surgery

rotation was a bore because the elaborate protocol and length of residencies means the neophyte student gets to do next to nothing in
eight weeks. He may hold a retractor or suture a few stitches, but
generally he spends long hours on his feet in sterile garb which prevents him from scratching an itch or retreating to the bathroom. The
student's interest in surgery is not improved by the early morning (6
A.M.) rounds or the second set of rounds in the evening.[2]

This bias against surgeons by third-year students with career
orientations in medicine is summarized in the following homily, told to
me by a third-year student:

> Psychiatrists know nothing and do nothing. Medicine knows everything
> and does nothing. Surgeons know nothing but do everything. Path-
> ologists know everything and do everything, but do it a day too late.

The key lesson of the third-year rotation or junior internship is
that the student learns the importance of management and all it entails:
(1) strategy, from history-taking to treatment; (2) plan of daily scut; (3)
reliance on consulting services, lab data, and so on; (4) the juncture
between the receiving ward and one's own service with regard to the
number and type of admissions;[3] (5) opportunities to discuss patients
other than one's own through the mechanism of rounds; and (6) development of clinical judgment. The third-year rotations are a concen-
trated effort in the internalization of the clinical perspective.

One of the ways the third-year student expresses his newfound
assertiveness is in his overt expression of preference for some kinds of
patients over others. The student no longer chastises himself for these
biases. In fact, the third-year student will think of these characteriza-
tions of undesirable patients as a kind of medical humor. This description of a "gomer" (sometimes called a "gork") is a classic:

> A gomer is your typical VA patient, who is seventy-five years old, has
> been smoking five hundred packs of cigarettes a year, has obstructed
> lung disease coming out of his nose, mouth, and lungs. He's a very
> whifty character who says "good morning, doctor" very, very slowly,
> such that you are gone from the room before he gets it all out.

Patients with psychological problems continue to rank poorly
in terms of desirability as patients. They occur across services, and
very few are ever referred to a psychiatrist, psychiatric social worker, or
psychologist. The population that is referred is likely to be in such
frank psychosis that psychological needs must be confronted. Unfor-

tunately, the probability of their improvement is marginal, compared to the prospects of moderately impaired patients who would be more likely to benefit from therapy. Such patients rarely receive psychiatric aid unless they themselves articulate the need for it. The "walking wounded" of psychiatry also include the professional patients, the "Munchausen," who present with classic symptoms and histories, often extensively rehearsed, knowing that their acts will bring admission.[4] There are also the "turkeys," the upper-class women who come into the hospital to rest from the burden of deteriorating marriages and senile husbands; the indigent, who want clean linen and some solid meals along with minimal management; the "sicklers" who are not in crisis; and the "sundowners." "Sicklers" are patients who suffer from sickle-cell anemia, a blood disorder characterized by recurrent painful attacks ("crises"). "Sundowners" are usually elderly patients with organic brain disease who become disoriented in the evening, when familiar surroundings take on an alien appearance and when loneliness and incapacity aggravate anxiety about dying.

By the student's third year, the definition of "the good patient" has expanded to mean a capable historian, who presents an organized and accurate history of the present illness and who is knowledgeable about past medical history. He seeks admission for "real" as opposed to "imagined" illness and has realistic expectations of the outcome of hospitalization. She or he is concerned about the nature of the illness and the required course of treatment, but is outspoken about neither the plan of treatment nor the expression of apprehension. The patient should be sufficiently verbal as to suggest the intelligence to comply with the doctor's orders, though evidence of having read up on the disease is generally greeted with coolness. It seems that patients who know the literature are under suspicion of emotional impairment until they prove otherwise. A woman who is well versed on her spouse's or child's illness is seen as a meddler and as neurotically invested in her dependents' illnesses.

A patient who distinguishes himself or herself by a pleasing personality (charm, wit, warmth, and capacity for gratitude) will be noted in the presentation of the case as, "Mr. Smith is a delightful man of seventy-two years, who presents with. . . . "[5]

Finally, the good patient does not make excessive demands on the physician for preferential treatment. "Political admissions" are patients admitted by high-ranking physicians, such as the chief of surgery, who require optimal patient-physician relations and top-notch nursing and related services. These patients often have more extensive stays in intensive care units than typical patients with the same condition. House staff repeatedly cited this as a major source of aggravation on services such as intensive care, where beds were in short supply. Political admissions entail elaborate series of phone calls from associates of the admitting physician informing house officers that they had better extend themselves for the duration of the political patient's hospitalization. Implicitly, such requests acknowledge variation in the quality of care within a given service at any time. There may also be tacit acknowledgment that such variation is morally wrong, but it is more commonly treated as an abuse of limited resources. Needless to say, patients who are identified as political admissions evoke much resentment from the staff.

It is curious that physicians who distinguish themselves as sources of "turkeys" and "political admissions" are tolerated as a necessary evil. House officers argue that their salaries are based on keeping the patient census high, and these physicians contribute to the hospital's economic solvency. Even though house officers complain about "Rosenberg's turkeys," they will do nothing to change his pattern of admissions.

The junior intern applies a more general rule of "not making waves," for when he does, he frequently gets in trouble. Yet the third-year student will venture a contradictory opinion when he feels he has ample grounds.

> Eddie Marx is a pediatric surgeon whose patient, Tommy Bennet, is a grossly retarded twelve-year-old boy. He has prescribed an antibiotic for Tommy, which the team of "Older Children-North" wants stopped because it may be masking infection, and Tommy has some fever. The use of antibiotics by surgeons is believed to be "dogma" and not rational procedure. Larry Renais, the third-year student, is sent to convince Dr. Marx to "d/c" [stop] the medication. He meets with no success. The resident goes after him and convinces Marx to stop it. Asked how he did it, he says, "Rationality."
>
> Two days later the cultures come back from the lab with ambiguous results. Only one of the two culture bottles grew out a positive culture. Larry talks the resident out of giving Tommy antibiotics. He argues that he would hate to put in an intravenous

line before the results are clear. An hour later Dr. Marx comes upstairs screaming, "Too many people are managing patients. The patient gets screwed. I'm running the show from now on." He chews Larry out, telling him that "to do a culture and ignore the culture is not a logical process." For good measure Dr. Marx lectures him on the cost of the cultures—$95 per test. Afterwards, Larry asks what he has done to deserve Marx's rage. "Cheer up," says the resident. "The next time he sees you, he'll greet you like an old buddy."

The third-year student will assert himself in other contexts as well. When one student learned of the possibility of getting a second asthmatic patient, when he really wanted someone with a different condition, he told his resident, "One asthmatic was fine, but Mr. Aspen is enough." The resident responded, "Give me some credit." The resident knows from his own experience that students seek out a variety of diagnoses in order to acquire a modicum of familiarity with the scope of "medicine." The third-year student will also suggest to his resident that he wants more responsibility and that he wants to know whether his current work is satisfactory. This contrasts clearly with the second-year student's passivity.

As the third-year student extends his boundaries, he is no longer intimidated by consulting physicians. He will actively seek their advice, which at times creates tension with the resident, who likes to minimize the number of people giving him orders.

Paul Harris, a resident, got angry with a third-year student when the student complained that he wanted a dermatology consult for a patient. "Why don't you worry about patients who are sick and quit futzing around," Paul retorted.

On the other hand, the third-year student will express his negative opinion of a consulting service. and thus justify his hesitancy in enlisting their help. Larry Renais hated to call in the neurologists during his month at Children's because after one or two unsatisfactory meetings with their attending physician, he decided that they act very serious and talk a lot in their special vocabulary; but they do not actually do much for the patients, and they hate to spend their time teaching students.

The third-year student no longer fears that each question he asks reveals the depths of his ignorance. He has acquired some basic confidence in his estimation of what a third-year student should know, and beyond that he simply wants to know as much as possible. A third-year student will exclaim, "What the hell is . . . ? I've never heard of it," without thinking it reflects on his inadequacy.

The one place the third-year student keeps quiet is with his advisor, when he goes in to discuss plans for his internship. Before going in to see his advisor, Larry Renais admitted, "My problem is whether I should be honest with these guys—if I should say, 'I just want to be Joe Blow in the community.' "

Tom Richards, his advisor, whose primary interest was research, kept emphasizing how University Hospital students land places in the best hospitals in the nation. He reported that he had been at hospitals in several other cities, as well as Children's, and that by comparison, Children's was "like a Sunday afternoon picnic." He commented that people at the VA enjoy a much calmer life-style, but without the institutional prestige: "Everybody there is happy as a fish. You must ask, 'What's it like at staff level?' " When Larry asked whether he should apply to children's hospitals or small hospitals, he was told:

Advisor: The former offer more mobility, both laterally and down. From Children's the only up is ——— Children's. With an M.D. from University Hospital you are eligible for a good internship. Try for the best, seek depth of training. . . . Keep a high profile and really work. Be aggressive, keep asking questions, tell them you want more patients. If I were you, I'd take an elective at my first-choice hospital. If this is a guy I know, I'll campaign for him because I'm dealing with a known. Plan for an October elective [an optional course or rotation].

Larry Renais was as low-keyed as University Hospital medical students come. When asked about how he copes with a slow rotation that prevents him from showing off his skills, he says, "You can't get upset about it." But throughout his whole interview with his advisor, he maintained the appearance of an aggressively compulsive University Hospital junior intern. The key point of emphasis—the development of his clinical skills—eclipsed any consideration of how he deals with patients as individuals or how he confronts questions of values in the practice of medicine.

One of the outcomes of the student's internalization of the clinical perspective is his need to push himself continually to see whether he can do a procedure without supervision and without running into trouble. He does have reservations about the limits of personal competence and expresses them in the following manner: "I don't want to do a femur stick without John [resident]. If you get in trouble, the patient could lose a leg. Such trouble is rare, but still I want him to know. She's bled out [She has no more usable veins]. Or he may ask himself how he can be ready to take on major-league responsibility when he still does dumb things like contaminate blood cultures through improper technique.

Sometimes he assumes a posture of having made a fatal mistake, when there is no reasonable basis for the assumption of culpability.

> David Hanson announced, "A monumental thing happened to intern David Hanson." He was referring to the death of his first patient. But he corrected himself and said that Mr. Giordano had been his first death, but it did not count since everyone had anticipated his death. "What I mean is Arnold Guest was my first unexpected death. As I was leaving Tuesday, the nurse asked me to listen to his lungs because they sounded congested. I concluded he had pneumonia. But Wednesday he was doing O.K. and had been sitting up in a chair. The resident and I went down to dinner, and when we returned we found him unresponsive. He had had an MI [heart attack], went into cardiogenic shock, and a code call failed to resuscitate him. Bill, the resident, said it took him an hour to track down the family because friends who had brought him in did not know the needed phone numbers."

In his concern for confronting what he should have done and in his need to review what had occurred, David Hanson absorbed some understanding of the probabilities with which physicians live. His anger had a quality of professional investment uncommon in the reaction of younger medical students. Paradoxically, this involvement elicited detachment.[6] This announcement was the only reference to the death of Arnold Guest that David volunteered.

David Hanson had a reputation among his peers for being exceptionally intense, earnest, and committed to academic medicine. In some ways he was the walking, talking, archetypal junior intern. At times he became so involved in the role of the "compulsive UH intern" that it was difficult to conceive that he might have a life outside the hospital. When he did go home, he reported, he would "pass out."

The position of the junior intern is highly ambiguous. He lacks the experience, skills, and authority of a genuine intern. Therefore, self-evaluation requires the juxtaposition of real and ideal standards of performance. In order to adjust for perceived inadequacy, there is a tendency to identify the ideal standards as illegitimate, but such a refutation is ultimately ego-damaging. It suggests that one is incapable of meeting universal standards of performance; and to do less than that is to subject patients to the risks of negligence and incompetence. While the third-year student will not analyze the situation in exactly these terms, there is the strong suggestion of such a legalistic perspective. In thinking of himself as a physician rather than as a student, the third-year student is forced to consider what the consequences are for the physician who fails to meet standards of professional performance.

The third-year student comes to feel that he is being held back from assuming responsibility for his patients, that he could take on more if he were not so highly supervised. He is prone to make remarks like, "Why are you studying how medical students acquire responsibility? They don't have any. You should go study interns."

In part he chafes because he is beginning to think of himself as a physician:

Junior intern (to a friend on gynecology): How do you like being a gynecologist?

Friend: Better than being, as you fellows say, "a physician."

Third-year student: So you're going into pediatric cardiology?

Fellow student: Yes, I don't want to be making $12,000 at age thirty. Now I'm not putting down the local peds—they have it hard.

The third-year student also begins to be treated like a "real doctor" by nurses and patients:

A former patient calls after "Dr. Renais" and the student confesses how exciting it is to hear his name spoken that way. "You know, he says, "this has happened just once before."

Nurse (to third-year student): I won't write the order because your resident is not here to co-sign it, but I'll talk to him about it.

Patient (to third-year student): You're gonna make a good little doctor because you're in earnest about what you're doing.

Student: That's neat.

By the last ten days of the rotation the third-year student is actively demonstrating that he is an intern. He questions management; he challenges the resident's recommendations. In an entourage he is in the vanguard, up close to the attending physician, rather than in the rear with the trailing second-year students and the head nurse who has decided to tag along. He has ceased to ask questions about the desired form of write-ups. He has acquired some familiarity with medications. He sometimes manages to be a step ahead of the resident in procuring lab data or requesting tests. While he has fleeting apprehension about making it as an intern, since it is a year-long proposition rather than four weeks, he has the necessary optimism that it will not be impossible to withstand.

After his junior internship, the third-year student will take "easy" courses for the next couple of months: rotations that require no nights and have regular hours. Courses like pulmonary medicine and dermatology fall into this category. If he finds himself in a boring course, like radiology, he will drop it without fear of recrimination. Other favored tactics are to elect "clinical holidays," two-week introductions to the clinical specialties of ophthalmology and otorhinolaryngology; the other possibility is to take an outpatient clinic course, such as outpatient medicine.

After his "vacation" he will tackle another junior internship, perhaps this time in pediatrics, in order to decide whether to apply for internships in medicine or pediatrics. If it is late in his third year, and if he has nearly all of his required courses completed, he may indulge himself with a month of real vacation.

The third-year medical student doing a junior internship is so concerned with keeping "on top of his patients" and securing an honors grade that he has neither the time nor the energy to indulge in moralistic thinking. Patients may die on the third-year student, but all he cares about is whether he contributed in any way to the patient's demise. The student is not concerned with whether the patient knew he was dying, suffered needlessly, or was afraid of death; nor does he worry about whether the patient should have been told earlier or more pointedly of the seriousness of the diagnosis. Nothing in his behavior would lead one to believe the third-year student is exceedingly callous or insensitive to suffering; rather, he cannot afford to worry about things over which he has little control. He must throw himself into what he can do for patients who are going to get out oï their sickbeds and go home cured, improved, or at least the same as when they came in.

The weekend after completing his junior internship, David Hanson called me and offered the following confession, which suggests that the ethical perspective is something of an afterthought once the immediate demands of the medical perspective have been dissipated: "I don't know if this is peculiar to me or more commonly experienced, but I've realized that in doing this course I lost sight of my goal. That is, to be the best goddamn doctor I can be, and do the best for my patients and never hurt them." He felt that he had been distracted from this goal by his preoccupation with getting things completed by a particular time, with the emphasis on citing the appropriate references. "In short," he concluded, "I thought what was important about this course was securing a recommendation for the best internship. I did not consider what that internship might mean in the light of these costs."

His self-evaluation contrasted with the evaluation of David's work by his resident, Bill Fleet. When house officers inquired about Bill Fleet, they always added, "Has anyone put him on Valium yet?" He was by reputation as well as by performance one of the most aggressive-compulsive, crackerjack residents in the house. Bill told David that he had done excellently as a second-year student, but had fallen short as a third-year student. He stated that he had inadequate knowledge of clinical subspecialties and that he failed to be consistently up on his patients. David asked him how well he thought he had managed his patients. Bill replied, "Excellent."

The third-year student has acquired some skills and some finesse. He is out to take on the stiffest possible demands to find out whether he will be able to function as an intern. An ill-timed word of criticism by an attending physician can throw the third-year student into a spasm of self-reproach and feelings of inadequacy; but a hint of praise can banish exhaustion, at least for the moment. For long stretches of time the third-year student neither eats nor sleeps. He merely lives on medicine. When he has completed this rite of passage, the third-year student knows he can survive all subsequent tests. Successful socialization means that the student has taken another step toward becoming "a real doc." And with hardly a pause to reflect, the student advances to the fourth year, secure in his acquisition of the clinical perspective of his superiors.

The third-year student has learned to use the clinical perspective as a way of alleviating anxiety over uncertainty and as a source of approval from his superiors. Rather than retreating into the moral perspective as he gains competence in his own judgment, he intensifies his use of the clinical perspective. Since he tends to think of himself as a physician, he also relies on the perspective of the physician as it is most commonly demonstrated—the clinical perspective. He rarely entertains the legal or moral perspective because he does not yet have any clear conceptualization of how they fit into the physician's role. While there is an occasional glimmer of recognition that both moral and legal considerations impinge on professional performance, they are not treated as directly relevant to being a physician.

10 The Fourth-year Student

Ask interns to name the best year of medical school or post-M.D. period, and they will tell you, "the fourth year of medical school." Some will admit that if there were such a thing as an ongoing fourth-year position with pay, they would sign on and forget the responsibilities of being a house officer. The high praise for this year is based on the fact that the fourth-year student is marking time till the M.D. degree and an internship in an accredited hospital. Until then, he occupies himself with "easy" courses, coast-to-coast trips to evaluate internship opportunities, a month or two of "real vacation," and an additional junior internship in an area of possible specialization. At University Medical School it is not uncommon for fourth-year students to finish up early and then take paid employment in area hospitals, such as City Hospital.

The fourth-year student bears little resemblance to the hyperactive third-year student. By now he has acquired needed recommendations for internships, has decided on an area of specialization, and has risen to a comfortable level in the status hierarchy. Through careful selection of rotations, the student has more time to spend on sleep and socializing. And professionally, the fourth-year student is equipped with enough self-confidence and clinical acumen to find clinical debate recreational, as long as he can score a point or two, based on demonstrating familiarity with the literature. And most important, the student begins to see the possibility of relaxing and taking things in, rather than constantly being on edge wondering what he should be doing, thinking, or reading, and how these performances will be evaluated.

When the fourth-year student elects a junior internship in such specialty courses as intensive care medicine or neonatology, he already has some inclination toward an area of medicine that will require these special skills. The student who elected the medical intensive care unit thought he would go into cardiology; the student who elected neonatology planned to specialize in pediatrics.

The kinds of courses fourth-year students elect assume basic competence of self-assurance. For example, in the medical intensive care unit one can ill afford to have a student who will need extensive coaching in the management of biochemical imbalances contributing to a comatose state. This assumption carries over into the utilization of consults. The student tends to apply a rule of self-interest whenever he is given some latitude: Will I learn something from the guy or will he simply create work for me? If the student believes the latter to be true, he will avoid taking the initiative to secure a consult, even though his resident may be admonishing him to call a consult "because at least you'll learn something from this patient." Quite frequently the implication is "Get a consult so that you'll learn something, even if it does not directly benefit this patient." To an outsider this use of patients as teaching material appears exploitative and unethical. To the house staff it is merely the means to an education.

The fourth-year student has become accustomed to games of probability, and he joins in the odds-taking, whether it be estimating bilirubin levels or wagering beers over the morbidity of a patient in intensive care. Anything that minimizes tension is appreciated, so the fourth-year student sees nothing "morbid" in guessing whether John Jones will "go down the tubes" while he is off for the night. As one student said, "Every time I decide to leave, John Jones goes and does something. All my patients die on me. Do you think he'll go before I come in in the morning? Any bets?"

While some of the excitement of medicine seems to have disappeared for the fourth-year student marking time in an "easy" course, there is always the possibility of landing a diagnosis that is a "zebra." Just after complaining about the lack of variety of patient complaints in University Hospital's emergency room, Chris Gorden got a fourteen-year-old black male with a complaint of hematuria (blood in the urine). After taking the history, doing the physical, and using the microscope, he turned and announced for my benefit: "A great case. Post-strep glomular nephritis. Wait till you see everybody turn around when I say that." The director of the emergency room examined the slide and was not convinced; he thought it was a simple urinary tract infection. The resident wanted a renal consult so Julia Marshall came down to look at the slide. She thought the boy should be admitted for observation and an extensive work-up because the clinic was inadequate for observation and follow-through. The boy was admitted the next day. Chris Gorden was very disappointed to learn two days later that the official diagnosis was "urinary tract infection."

Chris Gorden's delight in a serious diagnosis reveals the wedding of the clinical perspective to a subcultural value with ethical overtones (that is, an intellectual interest in clinical rarities is to be prized). This is different from the values of the second-year student in the early phase of clinical training. The neophyte second-year student hopes his patient will not be "really sick" or in pain. The perspective of the second-year student is a lot closer to the reality of the layperson than that of the fourth-year student. It is a reflection of different realities and their constituent values.

The fourth-year student likes to think of himself as a physician, while the reality constantly impinges on that assumption. For example, a 19-year-old woman came into the emergency room with a laceration on her calf that required stitches. Chris asked the intern what to do and was told to call the surgical resident, who gave him instructions. He was bending over the woman, slowly putting in stitches, when the intern came over to give advice.

Intern: The sutures should be small and close together because there's less scarring, and that's important to women, more so than to men.

Patient: It doesn't matter to me.

Intern: Then we'll sew you up with barbed wire because it's cheaper.

Three minutes later another intern came over to confer with Chris:

Second intern: Well, we just want him to perfect his job. There's nothing wrong with his work. We just want it to be perfect for you.

The surgical resident came along, looked at the sutures, and diagrammed their ideal placement. He sent Chris back to put in another two sutures.

The fourth-year student chafes under the institutional constraints which keep him in a closely supervised position. Increasingly he feels equal to those who must co-sign his orders:

Fourth-year student: Elmer [intern] is really hyper. He tells me I'm not supposed to make any decisions. I'm to ask him everything.

Other fourth-year student: It's really hard to be an intern.

Fourth-year student (to resident): Somebody technically has to sign this sheet. I have this guy with a sore throat. It's nothing to write home to mother about. Do you want me to culture his throat?

Resident: I don't care.

But by comparison with the second-year students, whom the fourth-year student observes doing their rotations, he realizes how much more freedom and responsibility he has. The second-year students serve as a negative reference group. He looks at these harried, seemingly lost students who need help starting intravenous fluids, who want to know how to ask the resident for a Saturday off, and he wonders how he ever endured the second year.

Teaching rounds are "no big thing" to the fourth-year student. He knows they are a means of reviewing patient management and resolving problems involving consult services, private attending physicians, and outside doctors. He takes them in stride, and his chief complaint is that rounds take too much time that he could better use doing scut.

Similarly, the elaborate art of scheduling has ceased to concern him. If he does not get the course he wants, he accepts his second choice and makes an agreement with himself that if it proves too boring or too much work he will drop it and spend the remainder of the rotation on vacation. And, like Alan Latrobe on psychiatry, if the course does not turn out to be what he wants, he begins to look elsewhere. Alan was supposed to spend eight weeks in the inpatient psychiatric unit, but the census was slow and his resident tried to hover over him. In the third week he announced that he had arranged with the chief of psychiatry at Community Hospital to take their psychiatric consultation course for the second four-week period. When his resident suggested that things might pick up and he would be given more responsibility, he failed to be swayed and left after four weeks.

The fourth-year student will not accept scut for the sake of doing someone else a favor, while in his younger years he would have been eager to help his intern either to earn good will or to acquire greater familiarity with laboratory techniques.

Resident: Are there any students interested in doing gram stains for T.B.?

Chris Gorden: I am the only student here and I am not interested.

Resident: I'll show you where the stuff is.

Chris Gorden: You have to be kidding. (He walks away.)

Out of sight of the resident, Chris roars at a re-creation of the scene: "Did you hear that guy? Did you see the look on his face when I refused? Just who did he think he is?" An intern, who has observed the whole scene, comes up to him and tells him to play it cool. "In the grand scheme of things, it doesn't matter much." However, Chris is still brimming over with a mixture of laughter and anger. He boasts, "This year I don't take any shit from interns . . . maybe residents. Last year I sometimes took shit, but not now."

By the fourth year, the student has dared to "fudge" data in order to spare himself excessive aggravation in dealing with the labs, which according to him are wholly inadequate and mismanaged. While the more junior student would feel obligated to explain an abnormal finding, even if it means entertaining an obscure diagnosis ("something as rare as rocking-horse manure"), the fourth-year student may look at an abnormal finding and ascribe it to "lab error":

Fourth-year student: These goddamn lab tests. You do the tests and get an abnormality, and you're stuck explaining it. . . . The hemoglobin on the first report was too high to be consistent with the rest of the data. I'll tell Mrs. J. she's in good health, that lab error held us up, and that she should come back to the ER [emergency room] if she gets dramatically worse.

The fourth-year student is no longer afraid to express un-equivocal disagreement with a house officer if he feels he has cause. The student will even go so far as to say, "I think I know about . . . , and I would recommend. . . . " George Smith, one of the least aggressive and competitive externs I observed, showed no hesitation in challenging his resident: George wanted to get an EEG (electroence-phalogram) of a female patient who had been having seizures since

4:30 A.M. The resident contended that it would not show anything useful that would affect therapeutic procedures.

George: The EEG will show a focus.

Resident: What is it going to show? She has focal seizures; this we know. If you want it, get an EEG.

George: It will tell us whether there is an electrical or anatomical defect.

Resident: An EEG won't tell you whether it is anatomical or metabolic.

George: Well, then it will tell you where the focus is.

Resident: It is unnecessary. We already know. . . . How much more exact can you be?

George: I'd rather do an EEG before I do an EMI [a very expensive and technologically complex brain scan].

Resident: I agree. I am not going to argue any more in front of our sociologist.

(The phone rang and it was the neurologist saying he wanted a stat EMI, which was scheduled for 1 P.M.)

The fourth-year student has mastered the classification of "turkeys" and "gobblers," and he applies the labels liberally to his patients. Patients who are not really sick are known as "turkeys," and "super turkeys" may be referred to as "gobblers." For example, a fifty-eight-year-old white female came into University Hospital with an admitting complaint of a bitter taste in her mouth and loss of appetite.

Intern: A turkey. Is she crazy?

Attending physician: What do you want to do?

Resident: Tell her barium is kind of soothing.

Student (as an aside): This is a real gobbler.

The mention of barium is a reference to a test that involves swallowing a chalky, highly unpleasant solution of barium for an upper gastrointestinal examination. Barium shows up as an opacity on the x-ray films. The pharmacist, in an aside, informed me that she had been admitted because her private physician is "high-ranking." He contended that 10 percent of the admissions to University Hospital were "turkeys," admitted because of politics. A common response to "turkeys" is to propose how one might punish them by causing undue pain or embarrassment. House officers also talk about doing the third rectal or pelvic examination, cutting off a "crust" (scab), or bronchoscoping, all of which are unpleasant or painful. The fourth-year student resents political patients because they take time away from "really sick patients." Regardless of the ridiculousness of a complaint, medical students (and their house officers) are obligated to check out all possibilities; some attending physicians would go so far as to advise repeating certain standard tests in order to avoid the possibility of a false negative.[1]

Some institutional settings intensify intolerance of "turkeys," such as the emergency room, where the short-term relationship between patient and physician removes the restraint that would be necessary in an ongoing relationship on a medical service. After seeing numerous patients with minor and often chronic complaints, the student loses patience and interest. In the intensive care unit or on the medical service, a patient with manifest psychological needs for hospitalization but without any organic basis for hospitalization evokes a kind of medical sarcasm which would horrify the typical layperson:

> Well, I guess it's time for his East Coast catheterization. After all, he hasn't had one for five years.
>
> What's the most painful kind of injection? Iron? Fine. How about daily iron shots for this lady.

Consequently, the fourth-year student looks in disbelief when the second-year student asks, "Aren't you going to do something about that lady's pain?" when the team has already decided she is a "turkey." He simply sees no reason to get excited about their blatant disinterest in her complaints and exudes an air of disgust with anyone who sees the matter differently. This exemplifies a latent concern with a moral perspective. Physicians place a value on treating "the sick" and consequently regard "turkeys" as a threat to their performance of that function.

Nearly every fourth-year student with whom I spent a rotation announced at the start that he would raise ethical questions. Just wait and see. With a certain degree of optimism I waited to hear him raise questions. But the fourth-year student is not concerned with ethical issues, because they rarely lead to a clear plan of clinical management. Another way of posing this bias away from ethical issues is to recognize that ethical issues in the clinical setting are frequently artifacts of procedures already entertained and executed on clinical grounds:

> Harry Fried [a fourth-year student] assisted Margey Ash [resident] in the delivery of a stillborn infant of a diabetic mother. Afterwards, as they returned to the nursery, Margey told him, "You know, I would have continued working on Baby Girl Marsh except Massenet [head of OB-GYN] told me to quit. He said there was nothing to do. As a resident it's tough to know when to quit."

Neither Harry nor Margey saw this as a question of euthanasia, the commitment of limited technological resources in a context of scarcity, or the obligation of the physician to limit heroics where "success" would mean a condition of lifelong idiocy (from brain damage) and dependency.

As the student comes closer to the realities of independent practice, he begins to give some thought to the legal implications of his responsibility as a physician. He knows about skull x-rays and taking spinal x-rays before giving shock treatments. He has seen several patients sign out against medical advice (AMA), so he is aware of the problem of liability. These realities are made concrete by notes on bulletin boards, like this one in the emergency room:

> If you advise a patient that a certain lab test or treatment is needed and he refuses, make him sign the AMA form. Unfortunately we're in the era where self-protection is essential. Do not let a patient leave against your advice without the AMA signature.

He also learns from his mistakes. In the emergency room, when the student gives a prescription for pills that the resident later notes should not be given to hypertension patients, he learns he must have the ward clerk send a letter of instruction to any patient released with an incorrect prescription.

In psychiatry, an area of medicine seemingly without a high probability of legal risk, the fourth-year student learns about "compensation neurosis," in which patients' mental problems exist concurrently with malpractice suits. He is advised against putting a certain patient on lithium, because "this is the kind of a guy who will sue you." A psychiatric resident lecturing on "how to commit someone" advises:

> With the recent furor over the rights of the mentally ill, you have to do an adequate job of "covering your ass." When you call that judge to ask for the commitment papers, you'd better tell a good story; and in fact, what you do is lie. On your first shot for commitment, you must get it approved—exaggerate if necessary. . . . I'm telling you that no, you don't have commitable grounds, but you have to sleep at night. Tell an exciting story. You had better make it convincing.

Harry Fried, a fourth-year student, was stopped one morning by the head nurse in the newborn nursery who wanted to know whether he had a consent for surgery form from the mother of a child with six fingers who was to have the extra finger removed. The surgeon would tie off the finger, which had no bone or nerves, and the finger would shrivel up and fall off. The look of surprise on Harry's face revealed his amazement that such a document must be secured. The nurse informed him that permits were required for this procedure as well as for a urinary catheterization and for a lumbar puncture (spinal tap). He was taken aback and asked why. She explained that it was because a needle is introduced into the body. When Harry asked how that differed from drawing blood, it was her turn to be speechless. She recovered to say that mothers sign a general consent form upon admission, which would cover the latter, but anything beyond this general set of procedures should be listed on a separate permit to protect the physician. She then admitted the infrequency of adequate consent. Harry could scarcely believe it: "Why, doctors would have to be followed around with secretaries to handle all the paperwork!"

Despite these experiences, the message does not quite hit home. The fourth-year student has little reason to see himself as legally vulnerable because he is protected by the intern's or the resident's signature. When Chris Gorden reported that a patient whom he had diagnosed as having a prostate condition turned up in the emergency room two days later with femoral thrombosis, a much more serious condition, Chris rationalized his mistake and did not express any recognition of possible legal consequences of this error in diagnosis: "Nobody had thought about it. The surgeon had come down and seen the guy and said he had prostatitis. He gave him an appointment in the urology clinic."

Medical students at University Medical School enter with the idea they will be survivors. The finale for the first-year students' "Freshman Follies," a spoof of the medical school, was "We Shall All Get Through," to the tune of "We Shall Overcome." They will endure what has to be endured in order to get the M.D., and then they will consider what else they want. This narrowly focused persistence can accomplish the task, but it can also lead to great disappointment. More than one house officer has expressed concern with why he or she has been willing to make so many sacrifices for this highly pressured, highly stratified kind of existence:

Harvey Gross (resident): I am not sure that this high-power academic medicine is what I want. Here you are nothing unless you've delved into the latest journals and maintained this intense relationship with medicine. I'm bored with medicine. You arrive at the end of a tunnel, and you find you know nothing about what lies outside of it.

Even the fourth-year student gets an occasional glimmer of what he has denied himself in order to get through. "Where are the role models," one student asked, "of physicians who have satisfying personal lives in addition to their professional performance?" Some fourth-year students seem to realize that some values have been lost or changed during medical school. The moral perspective, for example, seems to have gone underground. While it is conceivable that it may reemerge at a later time, there is a need for further research.

I have argued that ethical issues do exist in clinical practice but are only occasionally identified by students and house staff. More commonly, the student senses the ethical issues out of his overidentification with the patient, so that professional socialization, including the acquisition of "detached concern," reduces the salience of ethical issues. The more fully the student identifies himself as a physician, the more likely it is that ethical issues will be subordinated to clinical and legal issues. For the purpose of identifying and elaborating the nature of the three perspectives in medical training, I have treated them as distinct, while in practice they are frequently blurred. The application of these perspectives is most useful in showing the complex and interlocking nature of professional "reality," which is devoid of clear-cut boundaries.

Socialization to survival assumes an element of parsimony,

given the intrinsic simplification that occurs once the perspectives are ranked by frequency of use: clinical, legal, and moral. They are learned, however, in a different order: moral, clinical, and legal, thus, socialization necessitates repudiation of the perspective learned first. It would seem that medical students who survive medical school must make one of two choices: they must either minimize their ethical and legal perspectives in order to conserve mental and physical energy, or they must continually resolve the conflicts among competing perspectives by appealing to much more generalizable principles of action, such as the assumption that one can isolate "the interest of the patient." The latter alternative is clearly the more difficult to implement in terms of time and energy. In either case, the student must acknowledge that professional identity means change in oneself, whether actively pursued or passively accepted. A large component of that change is in the assumption of the clinical perspective, which appears to be part of self-definition by the completion of the junior internship.

As an intern once told me, medical school is training in anxiety and compulsion. Unquestionably, these two foci are stressed because they are the means to survival. In order to survive one must internalize the clinical perspective, for this is of paramount importance for acting like a physician. Only when one can identify the need for objectification, for the circumscription of concern, can one use both education and energies for the purpose of making patients better (or so students are led to believe). Regardless of the efficacy of clinical efforts, the fact remains that concern with ethical issues is treated as a holdover from a personal, nonprofessional perspective, which the student is not at liberty to support. The success of socialization is marked by giving up the ethical perspective in favor of the clinical and legal perspectives. As the student comes closer to independent practice as a physician, the salience of the legal perspective increases. I have also argued that by virtue of institutional placement and cultural and psychosocial identity, some attending physicians and house staff may be allowed to express concern with "ethical issues" beyond the scope of professional etiquette. But for the most part they are the exceptions, and the situations bearing recognized ethical issues are anomalies. The gradual ascendancy of the clinical perspective, the intrusion of the legal perspective, and the decreasing salience of the ethical perspective occur gradually and with some blurring, for neither the student nor his teachers and role models make clear distinctions between types of perspective or kinds of situations creating the need for their use.

In the next chapter the tension between delegation of authority and professional autonomy will be discussed as a means of opening up the problem of perspectives to the postgraduate years. It is a way of showing how ongoing socialization affects problem-solving; in particular, how institutional constraints on physician referral allow house staff to dispose of unwanted problems by passing them on to someone else. In some cases these "unwanted problems" contain some element of ethical concern. Consequently, we must ask, If physicians fail to assume responsibility for the acknowledgment and management of ethical issues in the clinical setting, to whom shall this responsibility fall?

PART FOUR

Social Policy Implications

11 Delegation and Autonomy: The Tensions of Giving and Taking

In this chapter the role components of delegation and autonomy will be examined in order to evaluate their contribution to the use of the clinical, legal, and ethical perspectives. Throughout professional socialization, physicians must come to terms with these interlocking facets of professional identity. Throughout their experiences in University Hospital, physicians decide which responsibilities they can give up to others without making excessive sacrifices in the quality of performance. This problem is common to all professionals who work with other professionals as well as nonprofessionals. For example, in the intensive care unit the chief respiratory therapist had primary charge of the calibration of the respirators, though students were frequently instructed in how to exploit the capacity of the machine. In the event of mechanical difficulty, the therapist rather than the pulmonary attending physician was called. Conversely, the physician must take up those aspects of performance which cannot be satisfactorily performed by others. At University Hospital only physicians were permitted to give certain very potent medications because the risks of incorrect dosage were too great to allow the responsibility to fall to the nurse. Both giving and taking responsibility are aspects of professional autonomy, which grants one the authority to make these choices. At the same time, the survival of the social institution in which these decisions are made depends on the internalization of an ethic of responsibility by its members. Regardless of whether one gives up or takes up a task, one is presumed to act with the interest of the institution in mind, rather than simple self-interest. Less abstractly, physicians may decide to delegate to medical students responsibility for patients; however, they (and their employing institution) are liable for

159

the consequences of the students' performance. While at times it may seem easier to the physician to do things himself, the overall goal of training physicians is better served through this type of delegation.

In the course of this chapter, I will argue that the problem of delegation goes beyond the allocation of clinical tasks to the delegation of ethical and social concerns. While the lay public has assumed that physicians should concern themselves with moral issues, there may be increasing room for nonphysicians to share in this responsibility. The fact that physicians are more likely to resort to the legal or moral perspectives when clinical options have been exhausted corresponds to their use of downward referrals in these instances. Thus, the internist refers his patient to the psychiatrist, or the psychiatrist elicits the help of the social worker.

There is reason to look beyond institutional constraints to the basic problem: How does one get physicians to give up tasks that could be adequately performed by less highly trained persons without having these physicians experience "role deprivation"? *Role deprivation* will be defined as the perception of a loss of self-esteem or status because a meaningful component of professional role definition has been lost through the delegation or usurpation of task function. For example, while students or house staff frequently attend routine deliveries, the obstetrician, in his interaction with the father, may still attempt to convey the impression that he has delivered the infant.

The use of midwives cannot become common unless obstetricians are willing to refer their routine deliveries to these practitioners and to occupy a role as supervising physician, available in the event of unforeseen complications. The attainment of this relationship would depend on the satisfactory resolution of the following questions: Would the obstetrician perceive a loss in self-esteem and professional status by working in close association with women (which most midwives are)? Would the physician be satisfied with a supervisory role in these deliveries, which would tend to make the patient less dependent on the physician, with primary loyalty to the midwife? Would the physician accept a loss of fees normally acquired through routine deliveries which would have to be compensated for through an increasing load of "problem" pregnancies?

This example, as well as the increasing utilization of social workers, physical therapists, lay therapists, and other ancillary personnel, requires the violation of a general rule of upward referral.

Normally, the house officer invokes the services of physicians of superior status when there is a problem in patient management, starting with the attending physician proceeding to the chief resident of a consultation service, and finally to the chief of the service. This referral is directed up through the status hierarchy. It minimizes uncertainty, for by having the opinion of one whose technical competence is highly regarded, the physician is bolstered in his use of the clinical perspective.

> When a ten-year-old white male came into the hospital with red mottled skin and high fever, the intern who admitted him could not construct a differential diagnosis that was adequate for the boy's condition. He conferred with the resident, who spoke with the attending physician. He suggested a consultation with the renal service. Eventually both the resident on call and the chief of the renal section came down to the floor to evaluate the case. After the diagnosis was made, and after extensive debate over surgery versus medical management, the surgeons were called in to offer their opinion.

In the event that the higher placed consultant should invoke the moral or legal perspective, the referring physician is likely to incorporate those perspectives into his or her own decision-making. Even if the referring physician (the subordinate) thinks the use of the moral perspective is highly idiosyncratic, he or she will probably go along with it because it is attached to a person of high status, which in itself is predicated on acknowledged clinical competence.

The relation of the physician to the nurse may be treated as a movement downward, but more significantly, the nurse fulfills the position of intermediary between the physician and assorted subordinate personnel. She may cajole the house staff into using the services of the dietitian, the social worker, or the clergy. She is the source of communication with the practical nurse, the orderly, the nurse's aide, and frequently the patient. This role is consistent with other situations of downward referral. The medical student is given duties at the discretion of the house staff; the student may be welcomed as additional help or disparaged as a burden on the unit. The third case of downward referral has to do with the status hierarchy within medical specialties. When all alternatives directed upward in the hierarchy have been exhausted, low-ranking specialists, most commonly exemplified by psychiatrists, may be consulted. The holders of this status are treated as so inferior that they can be called upon to do the unpleasant or to do what is perceived as an exercise in futility, such as finding a basis for unexplained somatic complaints or "curing" a postsurgical psychosis.

The relationship of the psychiatrist and the social worker is an interesting case of this problem of delegation and role deprivation. Compared to physicians working out of the emergency room and the general medical services, the psychiatrist makes the greatest use of the social worker. This is validated by the psychiatric social workers, who generally have worked in other in-house capacities before coming to psychiatry as a means of achieving greater professional autonomy. This autonomy is in part attributable to the frequent turnover in psychiatric house officers, so that the social workers must be relied upon to maintain constancy in staffing. Yet the psychiatrists whom I observed were very jealous of their own professional prerogatives and took frequent opportunities to denigrate the performance of the social workers. For example, meetings would be artfully scheduled to coincide with the social workers' obligation to be elsewhere. Nevertheless, the social workers, when interviewed, believed that their work was highly valued and that they were important to the functioning of the unit.

The sociological explanation of this antagonism is based on three principles of conflict. First, the psychiatrists on inpatient psychiatry were well aware of their inferior professional status, including their physical isolation from other medical services (they were housed in a building primarily devoted to private offices and the obstetrical services). Their inferiority was compounded by their reliance on the services of the social workers, who as nonphysicians contributed little to the psychiatrists' prestige. Psychiatrists never seem to overcome their status anxieties, which are initially identified as part of the student role, because their specialty has "low status." This seems to compound the onus of their close working relationship with social workers. It suggests that their colleagues view psychiatrists as "less than" regular doctors.

Psychiatrists have additional problems in dealing with delegation and autonomy because of their unique roles, which appear to affect their use of the three perspectives. While they are physicians and, thus, clinicians, their special skills involve "therapy." This commonly means that they receive patients after other physicians have failed, using the clinical perspective. Except when they make their own upward referrals to neurology and occasionally to "medicine," psychiatrists are generally cast in the position of accepting everyone else's failures. Their patients arrive on the service by virtue of acute crises which force referral by house staff who would prefer to contain the problem on their own services. Consequently, there is a relatively low success rate on the service, with many patients carrying histories of multiple admissions. Psychiatrists in this setting must therefore be able to get satisfaction from undramatic levels of improvement and management of chronicity —both low-status tasks in the university hospital. This tends to feed competition between psychiatrists and social workers for claims of improvement or "cure" which are necessary for professional self-esteem and consistent with the language of the clinical perspective.

When psychiatrists cannot sustain a clinical perspective, they may turn to a legal perspective rather than retreat to the moral perspective, which is closely identified with lay opinion. Therefore, it is not surprising that the legal perspective is used more frequently than the moral perspective by physicians on inpatient psychiatry.

In looking at the medical student and his socialization to delegation, we find a dual message: be possessive of those tasks which are clinically rewarding and divest yourself of those which are clinically unrewarding and those which are definitely legal or moral in their implications. The student hears his intern boast that he has not done a Wright's stain since his student days.* The student quickly learns that as a physician he may delegate the most unpleasant tasks: the postmortem care of bodies, any task related to bodily wastes, and the management of difficult, quarrelsome families. These kinds of tasks become the responsibility of the nurse, the nurse's aide, or the social worker. And as we have seen in diverse discussions, the use of consulting services is not highly valued, though some services are more respected than others. For the most part, it is something one is manipulated into doing—by the resident, by the attending physician, or by the exigencies of the case. Basically the student learns to be possessive of his responsibilities as they contribute to status. In some cases busyness is valued over and above the intrinsic significance of the component tasks. Students learn to feel guilty when they are not doing something, even while they are complaining that they do not have the time to think things through.

*A messy, time-consuming technique for preparing microscope slides.

It has already been suggested that not all the medical student's scut is dependent on a high level of skill and training. Part of the mystique of the physician is based on the layperson's lack of awareness of the low level of competence needed to perform basic scut, such as urinalysis. In fact, depending on the staffing of individual hospitals, medical students may find a varying proportion of these technical tasks delegated to nurses or special teams; for example, one may be able to pick up the phone and ask for the IV team, which is responsible for setting up the intravenous apparatus and maintaining it in good working condition.

When nurses have been trained to perform a large measure of the physician's scut, yet are forbidden to exercise these skills, they grow resentful. They openly complain that they are not allowed to do certain procedures because medical students need the practice. This, of course, is only the symptomatic expression of a graver condition. Skills are being wasted and sources of satisfaction are being denied for the sake of giving medical students responsibility for procedures of which they will divest themselves as soon as possible. Meanwhile, students are tied to these time-consuming tasks long after sufficient skill is obtained. The emphasis medical schools place on providing ample clinical experience for the student obfuscates the waste, inefficiency, and (unintended) discomfort for the patient. Here we see the ordering of the three perspectives in an institutionalized form.

While it is not commonly posed this way, returning the salience of ethical issues to the medical setting may necessitate reevaluating role definitions with respect to the delegation of duties. Throughout this book, physicians have been characterized as having tremendous authority and responsibility for patients' clinical well-being. In fact, when they have been criticized, it is because they appear to assume too much responsibility that might be delegated to others, professionals and nonprofessionals. For the most part, physicians base their authority in their clinical expertise, which allows them to weigh and evaluate objective, quantitative data in order to arrive at the treatment of choice. By thinking in this highly focused manner, physicians protect themselves from the distractions that would arise if they gave extensive thought to the numerous legal and ethical issues inherent in their decision-making. Generally speaking, they do not allow these other considerations to impinge on their clinical thinking unless there is some salient reason for opening up discussion to include such issues.

Second-year students do not see the wisdom of the defense mechanism until their attempts at survival are threatened. Their emotional investment in these auxiliary concerns is tacitly discouraged in order to force them to concentrate on clinical obligations. Without the prerequisite skills, these student physicians will not acquire the necessary foundation for patient-physician relations. Presumably, at a later time they may express their concern for "the whole person" of the University Medical School catalogue. For the interim, concern with ethical issues is implicitly delegated to other people.

This rationale could lead to charges of moral callousness and professional ignominy, to be corrected educationally.[1] The alternative position states the institutional bases for this behavior and suggests the need for utilizing supervisory and ancillary positions in the status hierarchy to allow physicians to confront the limitations of their professional role definition, at the same time freeing them from endlessly expanding responsibilities as the definition of normative behavior becomes larded with assorted "pastoral" duties. Specific suggestions along these lines will be set forth in the next chapter. Physicians viewed as technicians may have no greater claim to satisfying the interpersonal needs of patients than lawyers, and yet we are increasingly likely to demand such satisfaction from our encounters with physicians.[2]

The physician cannot consider delegation as a solution to increasingly complex role sets without autonomy derived from the institutional structure. Responsibility mediates between autonomy and delegation, however, as a condition of demonstrating power. This is true of informal relationships between physicians and other health-care workers. Where tasks are formally delegated on the basis of a strict status hierarchy, the discretionary power of the physician based on professional autonomy disappears. When hospitals, for example, routinely assign nurses the task of starting and maintaining IVs, the professional identity of the physician is no longer determined by a voluntary choice of performing or not performing in this capacity.

Autonomy consists of the authority to act independently or in conjunction with other health-care workers to fulfill role expectations. The authority to make such judgments distinguishes the physician from his or her subordinates. The nurse cannot usurp the prerogatives of the physician to administer medication or to start an IV but may assume these duties if formally requested by the physician. Similarly, the nurse has a degree of autonomy with regard to decisions to delegate tasks to the practical nurse, but the nurse is also expected to act responsibly, and to limit utilization of practical nurses to duties within their documented levels of skill.

More commonly, autonomy is discussed as the ability of physicians to do what they please, as long as it does not blatantly conflict with a professional code of ethics, such as the AMA Code, and as long as it does not displease a limited number of other physicians who act in supervisory capacities, such as chiefs of services. In other words, autonomy is a function of professional consensus, which is protected by the self-contained nature of professional circles.[3]

One consequence of sustained observation of professional behavior is the realization that the grounds of professional consensus are limited, even with respect to fairly objective situations like the appropriateness of a given antibiotic. The vast potential for conflict is mediated by the extensive professional autonomy granted to physicians by their peers, as well as by their patients. While there may be institutionalized means of review, such as the mortality committee which reviews all in-hospital patient deaths, or the patients' rights committee which is responsible for reviewing research protocols, most cases do not come under the review of supervisory agencies with any significant role in constraining physicians.

It is the naive belief of the layperson that a physician presented with a list of symptoms and a history of past and present illnesses, who performs a physical examination of the patient, can ascertain an unambiguous diagnosis and a course of treatment. Because of that assumption of omniscience, the patient adopts a passive role and allows the physician tremendous discretionary powers. Other physicians, who realize the nonrational elements in medicine, allow colleagues certain liberties as a means of recognizing "the art of medicine." Even when a colleague is clearly at fault, the bonds of fraternity are strong; each knows that his own professional identity may someday ride on the generosity of colleagues to cover up or defend rank incompetence. During the junior internship medical students learn the meaning of "covering your ass," and the lesson remains with them as their careers develop.

At University Hospital all charts are reviewed by the hospital utilization committee, which consists of former nurses who evaluate the charts with respect to length of hospitalization and appropriateness of treatment. When the projected length of stay expires, the committee reevaluates the chart and assigns a new projection. The intent of the review is to maintain optimal use of beds without keeping patients longer than is clinically necessary. Patients who are in need of long-term care can be referred to the social service department for possible nursing-home placement. The manifest reasons for chart review are circumvented by the purposeful creation of acceptable chart notes, that is, notes that justify extensions. The house staff writes notes that exaggerate the incapacities of a patient or elongate the progression of the convalescence if they have reasons for wanting that patient to stay. On the psychiatry unit, for example, patients' charts routinely carry grim notes of slow, almost imperceptible progress till the day before discharge. Then, miraculously, the patient makes a dramatic improvement that warrants immediate discharge. Such notes are justified by saying that insurance companies would not pay up if they thought a patient was well enough to go out on six-hour passes.

Malpractice is sometimes treated as synonymous with the abuse of professional autonomy. House staff at University Hospital, however, defined it as "faulty communication between physician and patient." Communication can continue between two people only as long as they share a common symbol system with identically ascribed meanings. There must be an element of complementariness in their relationship that allows each to listen while the other talks. The sequence of the thoughts of each must be comprehensible to the other. Patients and physicians start out with different vocabularies and frequently lack a basis for tying these two language systems together in a meaningful way. The physician may say, "Mr. Jones, you have a serious illness. We have found a malignant tumor on your esophagus"; yet the patient may not realize that he has cancer. Therefore, either the patient must find some way of unlocking the meaning of the physician's symbols, or the physician must step into the symbol system of the patient. The latter response contradicts the Weberian definition of "profession," which includes the use of specialized vocabulary and the possession of technical knowledge as a basis of professional identity.

The second means of managing the situation is to allow, in fact to encourage, the patient to ask questions and to become as involved in the discussion and management of his illness as he can. While physicians tend to be dubious about suggestions that patients may have a reasonable basis for participating in the treatment of their illnesses, they are eager to achieve patient compliance. It may prove sufficient for the physician to offer the patient the opportunity to discuss the regimen and its associated problems with a nurse-practitioner or other ancillary professionals. Physicians frequently prejudge their patients by their education and income to determine whether they have the ability to absorb medical information. They also fail to recognize the highly technical level of the information extended to the patient, even when they think they have simplified to the point of exhaustion of information. The problem of translation into the vernacular is basic. When patients feel they have been unfairly excluded from discussion of their illness and feel they have no way of redressing their powerlessness because the physician cannot translate the problems into a common tongue, they may take their cases to the courts on the issue of "informed consent" and express their dissatisfaction in moral rhetoric. A recent study has concluded that the highly trained physician who practices in a hospital setting is the usual defendant in malpractice suits, implying that incompetence is not the basis of the initiation of claims.[4] Nurse-practitioners may be able to provide a valuable service by acting as "medical translators" between the patient and the physician. They may bridge the disparate realities and increase patient satisfaction with medical services. Autonomy in and of itself may offer a less satisfactory explanation of the increase in malpractice litigation than the house officers' explanation based on communication; yet in their own handling of patients, they tend to go after the extra x-ray rather than the additional minutes of conversation with patients.

The two issues of delegation and autonomy come together in the increasingly public sphere of the practice of medicine, which has the effect of contracting the sphere of professional autonomy. The practice of medicine has come increasingly into public view through the greater clinical sophistication among laypersons born of *Readers' Digest,* television, health commentators, campaigns by different societies (such as multiple sclerosis and cancer), and television dramas which portray symptoms of rare diseases; the greater need for record-keeping and other forms of documentation which then become subject to the review of nonphysicians, such as insurance companies and utilization committees; and the greater incidence of malpractice suits.[5] Once there is awareness of potential culpability in physician performance, awareness of error also intensifies. A fourth consideration is the change in the social relationship between patient and physician. The physician is no longer on intimate terms with patients and their families, and thus there is no emotional bond which would require patients to keep the relationship "private." There is no longer any reason to protect the reputation of the physician, nor is there any reason to trust his or her implicit judgment. Where the physician is forced to spell out the rationale for treatment, an intrinsically private relationship becomes public.

The increasingly public sphere of the practice of medicine is typified by changes at both ends of the life cycle. The frequent attendance of husbands at the birth of the child, and the transition from the home to the hospital room as the place of dying, mean that one comes into the world and exits from it in the public eye. Questions about the subtle distinctions between "passive" and "active" euthanasia are instances of the examination of an informal practice that has now become open to scrutiny. The formal articulation of rules of performance may prove more difficult to enforce effectively than has been foreseen, or more cruel in their consequences than was anticipated. Just as the articulation of aesthetic criteria cannot create a work of art that is universally recognized as a masterpiece, so the espousal of criteria for the salvageability of a life cannot fully connote the meaning of that fragment of life to the person in question.

The constraint of professional autonomy by public observation minimizes the arbitrariness in professional practice. There is a recognized need for the laity to affect medical practice in ways that will preclude the possibility that "codes" will be called on the basis of who is on call for the night, or the chance that unnecessary surgery will be ordered for the sake of lining the physician's pockets. But it is a dual-edged sword which requires both patients and their physicians to take responsibility for their medical care. For example, when women request "family-centered" deliveries, where husband and friends participate in the birth, they limit the discretionary power of the obstetrician or midwife to deny the newborn the means to survival, if upon initial examination the newborn proves to be grossly defective. With witnesses to the live birth, the physician or midwife is not going to risk a malpractice suit for the sake of sparing the family the lifelong burden of caring for this defective infant. The responsibility falls to the husband and wife to discuss, in advance of the birth, their wishes under such conditions—or suffer the undesirable consequences. In fact, I would suspect that in this hypothetical case, the burden of bearing and caring for this defective infant would feed any latent distrust or dissatisfaction with the birth attendant, contributing to the possibility of a malpractice suit. This is the reverse of the intended consequence of the action to sustain the life.

Patients may contribute to the physician's disregard of the moral and legal perspectives by their willingness to hand over full clinical responsibility—"cure me." If they grant physicians unlimited autonomy as a condition of their professional relationship, they must generally take the consequences of that professional paternalism. If physicians will not accept the patient's claims to a share in the responsibility, the patient must either educate the physician as a condition of continuing the relationship or seek another physician. Patients may play an important function in persuading physicians to delegate facets of their roles to other health-care workers by demanding referral to nurse-practitioners, social workers, or the nutritional services of a hospital department of dietetics. Similarly, they may identify ethical and legal issues and bring them to the attention of physicians.

The two opposing terms of professional identity, delegation of roles and autonomous performance, are manipulated by physicians in their efforts to deal with the three perspectives we are examining. When clinical judgment fails to resolve a clinical problem, physicians are likely to delegate the problem to subordinates who, in conjunction with their low status, may be inclined to use the legal or moral perspective. When physicians think that clinical problems can be resolved by use of the clinical perspective, they may assert their autonomy and assume total responsibility for the patient. In the numerous situations where the effectiveness of the clinical perspective is uncertain, there may be much "punting" (passing the buck) and "waffling" (equivocating) as decisions are passed from person to person within the status hierarchy, though the general pattern is upward referral.

In the course of their socialization, students are explicitly taught that autonomy and the assumption of clinical responsibility are important attributes of the physician. But implicitly they are shown that these two elements of role definition are not sufficient to resolve clinical problems with legal or ethical components. Resolving these problems is treated as a dilemma because physicians continue to see the solutions resting exclusively with themselves. Delegation of responsibility, including legal and moral responsibility, may contribute to the resolution of the tension between giving up and taking on responsibility as the basis of professional identity.

12 Conclusion

The identification of three perspectives in the clinical setting illuminates the complexity of clinical reality as it impinges on physicians in decision-making capacities. While a review of the sociological literature of the late 1950s and early 1960s suggest a lack of concern with ethical issues among medical students and their role models, more recent publications and my own university experiences had led me to believe in the existence of a new kind of medical student who, encouraged by his or her teachers, actively pursued discussion of ethical issues. Extensive participant observation in a university teaching hospital failed to substantiate these assumptions. Instead, I found that medical students are being socialized into using the clinical perspective to resolve clinical problems with little or no regard for the ethical aspects of their professional behavior. In particular, there is a striking absence of both discussion of and concern with ethical issues, despite a growing body of literature that argues for the relevance of training in ethics for physicians in an age of technological medicine.

The three perspectives in the clinical setting are the clinical, the legal, and the moral. The clinical perspective entails the evaluation of patient history and physical examination, laboratory data, and available consultants' reports; together they create "the clinical picture." It is supported by access to medical literature and the accumulation of clinical experience. The use of the clinical perspective results in the development of "clinical judgment." The legal perspective entails evaluation of the facts of a case, the citation of relevant case precedent, and the search for additional legal principles that might contribute to new interpretations of the law. When the legal perspective becomes relevant to clinical decision-making, the introduction of clinical evidence serves as an effective constraint on the applicability of the law. The necessity of "expert medical testimony" as a condition of judicial consideration tends to support the use of informal procedures in order to minimize the need for court opinion. Physicians do not like to testify against each other, nor do they like the possibility of court intervention in clinical practice. In the event that the court intervenes to resolve questions of professional judgment, whether through a court order or a trial, the burden of evaluation of the clinical evidence rests with non-physicians, the judge or jury. The use of the legal perspective results in "legal judgment." The moral perspective entails the evaluation of available data to determine whether an action meets the standards of personal value judgments and thus, is desirable. It consists of judgments of "right" and "wrong."

It is possible to rank the three perspectives in the clinical setting. These rankings vary with the institutional status of the decision maker. Each of the following orderings is the most general case for the given institutional status: (1) Medical students, upon entering University Medical School, use the moral, the clinical, and the legal perspectives, in that order. After acquiring clinical experience, they apply the ranking of physicians. (2) Physicians use the clinical, the legal, and the moral. (3) Hospital administrators invoke the legal, the clinical, and then the moral. (4) Laypersons use the moral perspective and depend on professionals to provide the clinical and legal perspectives, though they may use information from the media in an attempt to address the clinical and legal aspects of problem solution.

Although distinctions among the three perspectives are not always clear-cut, the clinical and legal perspectives tend to be characterized by principles of objectification, concreteness, and case-by-case review. The moral perspective, in contrast, is characterized by subjectivity and diffuseness. All three perspectives are subject to the effects of social change, and thus are distorted if we conceptualize them as fixed entities.

Furthermore, no single perspective is solely in the hands of one profession or one category of individuals. Physicians do consider the legal consequences of their actions, and lawyers must evaluate clinical evidence in order to prepare a brief in a malpractice case. Nevertheless, the clinical perspective prevails in the problem-solving of physicians, just as the moral perspective prevails in the problem-solving of laypersons faced with a medical decision.

While it has been the thesis of this book that physicians employ the legal or moral perspective only after they have exhausted the clinical perspective, clinical situations have been noted in which physicians have acknowledged ethical issues in conjunction with clinical judgment. The rarity of these situations, however, has led me to characterize them as anomalies. Both the presence and the absence of the ethical perspective have been explained on the basis of institutional constraints, role demands, and psychological factors.

It is in the examination of socialization to survival, the professional socialization of second-, third-, and fourth-year medical students, that the ascendancy of the clinical perspective has been illustrated. While role models do exist who stress the needs of "the whole patient" and related ethical issues, they do not seem to be perceived as desirable models.

During medical school the students learn to identify the assumption of responsibilities with acting like a physician to such an extent that it is difficult, later in their training to give up responsibilities to others in the status hierarchy who might be equally capable. The responsible delegation of tasks might also include the delegation of responsibility for the psychological and social needs of the patient. In particular, people other than the primary-care physician might be given responsibility for identifying and responding to the ethical aspects of clinical care. In consultation with the primary-care physician, ancillary staff might contribute to the program of clinical management by clarifying these concerns. There seems little justification for the assumption that physicians *qua* physicians should have the inclination and the skills to address ethical issues in clinical practice. In fact, a constellation of factors (such as time, status, and personality) work against such considerations on the part of the physician. Physicians are burdened by culturally sanctioned role definitions as well as institutional constraints that impinge on their clinical decisions. This is most commonly expressed in the system of referrals and the solicitation of consultations. They also lack the time and energy to make a greater personal investment in the ethical and legal perspectives. However, as the possibility of lawsuits becomes increasingly real, physicians may be expected to use the legal perspective more often.

In looking at the tension between autonomy and delegation as it affects the use of the three perspectives, I have argued for the need to recognize the social stratification within university teaching hospitals as well as the hierarchical structure of the medical specialties. I have argued for the need to delegate authority to subordinates in the hierarchy when they can perform the duties that physicians have assumed without reducing the quality of care. Moreover, by increasing the delegation of tasks, physicians would free themselves to do those tasks which others in the status hierarchy cannot perform. In essence, physicians must learn that delegation is not tantamount to irresponsibility. What is needed is the responsible exercise of professional autonomy, which allows a physician to clarify the parameters of a task and to assign it to the appropriate subordinate when the physician is not assumed to be irreplaceable.

While it is outside the scope of this book to discuss the possible utilization of physician extenders, including the corpsman, the nurse-practitioner, and the physician-assistant, the problem of delegation affects all of these potential members of the health-care team, especially since physicians seem hesitant to avail themselves of these assistants.[1] A whole new aspect of technical assistance could grow out of the use of nonprofessional aides who might be given the general title of "peer counselor."

In a variety of settings, patients need emotional support that ranges from daily visitors, to advice on dealing with the limitations of chronic dialysis, to assistance in eating and with small chores like mailing a letter. While there has been some attempt to make nurses more sensitive to patients' needs in these areas, and much criticism of physicians for failing to address the nonclinical needs of patients, doctors and nurses are not ideal candidates for roles of counselor, confidant, and friend.

The following possibilities illustrate how the problem of delegation could lead to the use of laypersons to free the technically skilled professional from misusing time and skills that other health workers do not possess.

1. The intensive care nursery could benefit from nursery "grandmothers" who could informally talk with mothers (and fathers) who are terrified of their incompetence in handling, feeding, and caring for their premature or sickly infants. Many of these people have become parents for the first time and lack experience with infants, so that the simplest operation, changing a diaper, becomes a challenge to their competence as parents. They may be hesitant to ask nurses their questions because they fear they will be thought stupid, while physi-

cians complain about their exhaustive lists of insignificant problems. Frequently the nursing staff lacks sufficient time to encourage new parents to voice their questions.

2. Patients who are candidates for surgery frequently suffer from exaggerated fear of the procedure, sometimes to the extent that they will refuse needed surgery. These fears could be at least partially alleviated by talking with someone who has undergone similar surgery. Patients with chronic incapacities need the opportunity to talk with someone who is aware of the ramifications of their illness on relationships with friends and family. The counseling of mastectomy patients by other women who have had mastectomies is the prototype of peer-to-peer counseling.

3. Patients who experience abandonment by their families or geographical separation from potential visitors often make additional demands on the medical staff as an expression of their unhappiness. Professional "kibbitzers," people who would visit patients regularly for the sole purpose of conversation and a show of concern, would improve patient morale and have the latent function of decreasing demands on nursing staff for attention.

Obviously, such needs arise from the absence of other resources, such as the family. It is another example of how the failure to satisfy private needs through personal resources creates the desirability of a public solution. Yet what is to be considered in the light of this transformation is who should fulfill these needs and by what means. The expansion of the physician role is one possibility; the careful use of subordinate personnel has been suggested as a more reasonable alternative.

Such support roles would require a highly developed system of volunteers or the availability of funding to pay for these services, which would probably fall into the category of supplementary income for the elderly or for those who can only work part time. Nonetheless, in our absorption in the increasingly technological aspects of medicine, we forget that the inherent dysfunctions of this highly impersonal, objectifying form of medical practice may be redressed by people other than the physician. The formal delegation of those tasks which were previously undefined and allocated by default may increase the efficiency of the physician and the satisfaction of the patient.

One test of the richness of research is the manifestation of additional research queries. The research implications of these findings are many. They can be divided into further research in applied sociology and further research in theoretical sociology.

The following questions need to be raised within applied studies:

1. What is the long-term effect of university medical training? Graduates of university teaching hospitals who do residencies in community hospitals may make greater use of the ethical perspective than do their peers who select residencies in university settings. It would be important to follow these graduates five and ten years after the completion of their residencies to determine whether the residency site affects the use of the ethical perspective. Another way of looking at this question would be to provide the same case histories to physicians trained in university hospitals, using samples of house officers and doctors with five, fifteen, and twenty-five years' experience in the university setting, to see whether there is a subsequent emergence of the ethical perspective.

2. What is the effect of institutional status on the use of the ethical perspective? Within university teaching hospitals it would be helpful to see whether institutional status is a predictive factor in the use of the ethical perspective. The use of social factors in clinical decision-making might also be explored. Samples should be taken from chiefs of services, attending physicians, and house officers. A second set of samples might be taken from representative specialists to see whether some kinds of specialists are more disposed to use the ethical perspective than others.

3. How do female physicians compare with their male peers in the relative use of the clinical, legal, and moral perspectives? With increasing numbers of women attaining admission to medical school, some people have argued that the presence of women will "humanize" medicine. Given the same case histories to evaluate, do female physicians make greater use of the ethical perspective than their male peers? If there is a significant difference in the relative weighting of perspectives, it could affect those specialties in which women are more numerous, such as pediatrics and internal medicine.

4. Are physicians more inclined to define male malingerers as "Munchausen" and female malingerers as "turkeys"? The identification in the medical literature of professional patients, "Munchausen," suggests a degree of clinical objectivity not conveyed by derogatory terms such as "crock" and "turkey." While the existing literature does

not make any clear case for the assignment of "Munchausen" by gender, the sexist bias of physicians in the university hospital setting suggests that women may be more likely to be characterized as "turkeys" than as "Munchausen," even when they present a history and related complaints comparable to the rehearsal and performance of genuine Munchausen. To study this question, half the sample of physicians could receive a case history labeled "female" and half the same history, labeled "male." Furthermore, the population of physicians could be divided into male and female and all possible combinations accounted for: male medical doctor and male patient, male medical doctor and female patient, female medical doctor and male patient, and female medical doctor and female patient.

Several possibilities for research in theoretical sociology also exist:

1. In prior chapters of this book the local physician, the second-year student, and the physician who gets sued have all been treated as negative role models. Within role theory there is need for further elaboration of the meaning and significance of negative role models. The concept of "role deprivation" has also been introduced in conjunction with "role loss" and "role sets." The literature on life cycles includes discussion of role loss in retirement and of women's role loss with the departure of the last child from the parental home. Yet these are situations over which the individual has very little control. In the context of physicians delegating authority to subordinates and experiencing role deprivation, I have been speaking of a conscious choice. Where institutional constraints require delegation, as in the use of teams, I would argue that physicians experience role loss. But where they give up a role with hesitancy and displeasure, I would explain it as role deprivation. For example, psychiatrists give up some aspects of family therapy to the psychiatric social worker; however, they may obstruct the social worker's efforts to fulfill that delegated responsibility. The subtle differences in the two concepts may be useful in talking about illness behavior and patient compliance, as well as about political leadership and social change. Conceivably people respond differently when they perceive depletion of their role sets as role loss as compared to role deprivation. There may be another distinction requiring a third formulation of role loss, "role refusal." A role may be available to a person but not incorporated into his or her role set through conscious or unconscious rejection of it, for example,

when a wife refuses to accept the "mother" role in her relations with her husband, or when she declines the role of "a sister" vis-à-vis her daughter.

2. The specialized vocabulary of university house staff, such as, "gobblers," "red snappers," and "gomers," is an extension of ideology. Further study is needed in the development of language as a means of expressing and maintaining an ideological position.

3. The idea of three perspectives, at times competing and at times complementary, requires broader theoretical exploration of the nature of multiple realities. Within the sociology of knowledge it is common to speak of the problem of "consciousness" as both ideological and structural. What is the relationship of multiple perspectives to professions in general? By virtue of professional expertise does one confront multivalent criteria for decision-making? And if so, what are the sources of related perspectives?

The generative capacity of the idea of multiple perspectives in decision-making leads to a richness of research potential. In the course of my research the negation of initial assumptions has produced a complexity of issues. The ascendancy of the clinical perspective in the training of physicians and the practice of medicine may be an artifact of cultural lag. Perhaps physicians have not yet realized the importance of enumerating the ethical as well as the legal aspects of clinical problems, though the technological basis for such concerns already exists. Regardless of the likelihood of remediation, laypersons concerned with these issues must acknowledge the constraints on medical practice. For without recognizing the discrepancy between the layperson's depiction of the clinical reality and the physician's, the possibility of finding a common ground is very small, and the potential for antagonistic relations is very great. The respective problems of patient and physician are not going to be resolved by the assertion that one conceptualization of reality is superior to the other. They will remain different depictions of a commonly identified reality. What may be found are ways to exploit common needs and interests and to satisfy them by expanding professional delegation of authority.

Two broad social changes in the relationship between the medical profession and the lay public are the increasingly public sphere of medical practice and the increasing medicalization of social life. Public outcry and dissatisfaction with the abuse of autonomy by physicians is an expression of the desirability of public solutions for private problems. Impaired patient-physician relations are no longer seen as a private concern between patient and physician. Similarly, public dissatisfaction with increasingly high rates of social problems has contributed to the transformation of social problems (alcoholism, deviance, promiscuity) into medical problems in order to exploit the powers of physicians as curers and healers. This is a double bind. On the one hand, the public complains that physicians have too much autonomy and power; on the other hand, they rebuke them for their unwillingness to assume responsibility for the problems the public would gladly dump at their feet.

The moral rhetoric of the angry public exemplifies the use of a single perspective, the moral perspective, to approach complex problems that require the use of the clinical and legal perspectives as well. Because the public lacks the professional expertise of physicians and their lawyers, they are left to argue in moral terms. While many have argued that change must come from physicians, there is no reason to believe that change cannot come from a public that is becoming increasingly equipped to express its needs as health-care consumers. With the increasing sophistication of patients and their representatives, laypersons may be able to break down some of the mystique of physicians. In doing so, they will increase their autonomy while improving the quality of health care. At the same time, physicians will be relieved of some of the responsibility that comes of professional paternalism and the assumption of their irreplaceability. Eventually physicians may be limited to their roles as diagnosticians and technicians in an era of medicine where technology rules. Should this happen, their own confusion with the ethical aspects of medicine will be returned to its rightful place: the concern of men and women in the twentieth century with the quality of life.

Notes

Preface

1. Dr. Renée Fox, *Experiment Perilous: Physicians and Patients Facing the Unknown* (Philadelphia: University of Pennsylvania Press, 1974; first printed by the Free Press, 1959); idem, "Training for Uncertainty," in *The Student-Physician,* ed. Robert Merton, George Reader, and Patricia Kendall, 2d ed. (Cambridge, Mass.: Harvard University Press, 1969).

2. Renée Fox, "Is There a 'New' Medical Student?" *The Key Reporter* 30 (Summer 1975), 2.

3. The Hastings Center (Hastings-on-Hudson, N.Y.) was founded "to fill the need for sustained, professional investigation of the ethical impact of this biological revolution." The institute has three goals: "advancement of research on the issues, stimulation of universities and professional schools to include ethical inquiry as part of their curricula, and public education" (From Statement of Purpose by the Institute).

4. Elizabeth Kübler-Ross, *On Death and Dying* (New York: Macmillan, 1969).

5. The major bibliographic source is a serial publication covering articles published since 1973, published by the Kennedy Institute for the Study of Human Reproduction and Bioethics: *Bibliography of Bioethics,* ed. LeRoy Walters (Detroit: Gale Research, 1975-). A more accessible source is James Carmody, *Ethical Issues in Health Services: A Report and Annotated Bibliography,* (Washington, D.C.: U.S. Department of Health, Education, and Welfare, 1974).

6. For discussions of ethnomethodology see Harold Garfinkel, "The Origins of the Term 'Ethnomethodology'," in *Ethnomethodology* ed. Roy Turner, (Baltimore: Penguin Books, 1974), pp. 15–18; and Harold Garfinkel, *Studies in Ethnomethodology* (Englewood Cliffs, N.J.: Prentice-Hall, 1967). For a history of the development of ethnomethodology as a research method, see Colin Fletcher, *Beneath the Surface: An Account of Three Styles of Sociological Research* (London: Routledge and Kegan Paul, 1974), pp. 105–107. A more general reader, *Recent Sociology, No. 2,* ed. Peter Dreitzel (New York: Macmillan, 1970), is also useful.

7. See George McCall and J. L. Simmons, *Issues in Participant Observation* (Reading, Mass.: Addison-Wesley, 1969); as well as Leonard Schatzman and Anselm Strauss, *Field Research: Strategies for a Natural Sociology* (Englewood Cliffs: Prentice-Hall, 1973).

8. The two classic works are Merton, Reader, and Kendall, eds., *The*

Student-Physician, and Howard Becker et al., *Boys in White* (Chicago: University of Chicago Press, 1961).

9. Harold Becker, "Problems of Inference and Proof in Participant Observation," *American Sociological Review* 23 (December 1958), 652-660; Merton, "Field Work Evidence," in *The Student-Physician,* pp. 39-62.

10. The problem of ethics of research, including the problems in the publication of field studies, has not been addressed. For an article which elaborates on these problems, see Paul Reynolds, "Value Dilemmas in the Professional Conduct of Social Science," *International Social Science Journal* 27 (1975), 563-627. Other sources are Howard Becker, "Problems in the Publication of Field Studies," *Reflections on Community Studies,* ed. Arthur Vidich, Joseph Bensman, and Maurice Stein (New York: John Wiley, 1964) pp. 267-284; Clifford Geertz, "Thinking as a Moral Act: Ethical Dimensions of Anthropological Fieldwork in the New States," *Antioch Review,* 28 (1968), 139-158; Lee Rainwater, and David Pittman, "Ethical Problems in Studying a Politically Sensitive and Deviant Community," *Social Problems* 14 (1967), 357-366; and Arthur Vidich and Joseph Bensman, *Small Town in Mass Society,* rev. ed. (Princeton: Princeton University Press, 1970), pp. 397-476.

Introduction

1. The two classic sociological studies of the professional socialization of medical students are Robert Merton, George Reader, and Patricia Kendall, eds., *The Student-Physician* (Cambridge, Mass.: Harvard University Press, 1969); and Howard Becker et al., *Boys in White* (Chicago: University of Chicago Press, 1961). A review of the professional socialization literature is found in Agnes Rezler, "Attitude Changes During Medical School: A Review of the Literature," *Journal of Medical Education,* 49 (November 1974), 1371-1375.

2. Samuel Gorovitz and Alasdair MacIntyre, "Toward a Theory of Medical Fallibility," *The Journal of Medicine and Philosophy,* 1 (March 1976), 51-71.

3. See Eric Cassell, *The Healer's Art* (Philadelphia: J. B. Lippincott, 1976) for discussion of this orientation to medical practice.

4. Charles Fried, *Medical Experimentation* (New York: Elsevier, 1974).

5. Cf. Gorovitz and MacIntyre, "Toward a Theory of Medical Fallibility," p. 55.

6. Eric Cassell, "Moral Thought in Clinical Practice: Applying the Abstract to the Usual," in *Science, Ethics and Medicine,* ed. H. Tristram Engelhardt, Jr., and Daniel Callahan (New York: The Hastings Center, 1976), pp. 147-160.

7. Fried, *Medical Experimentation.*

8. In *The Healer's Art* and other writings, Cassell argues, (and he would be supported by many) that the task of the physician is to be both healer and curer. From Cassell's own writings, it appears that he has made this synthesis and he is scornful of the new, young doctors who fail to achieve this model of performance. Indeed, he seems to suggest that if he and others of his generation could do so, why not these physicians? Even if we would wish to accept his argument that experience is the great mellower and source of humility, we would have to acknowledge that the present generation of physicians is acquiring sets of experiences radically different from those of their mentors. I doubt that these younger physicians can achieve Cassell's ideal

within the university research setting. Indeed, it is time to consider whether this is the appropriate setting for all medical education, regardless of ultimate specialty, including primary care.

9. René Dubos, *Mirage of Health* (New York: Harper and Row, 1959), pp. 129–169. Hygeia was the goddess of health, a guardian of the sick. She was the embodiment of rational living as a condition of maintaining physical and mental well-being. Asclepius, the first physician, according to Greek legend, became famous because of his skills with a scalpel and his knowledge of curative plants. Asclepius thus represents the treatment of disease through specialized knowledge.

10. For example, a patient on the psychiatric service suffered from severe depression. According to her history it was related to an automobile accident in which she had been injured. A closer examination of the story revealed that about that same time her husband became dependent on kidney dialysis. When I pointed out the convergence of the history and elaborated on the social factors of chronic dialysis, the attending physician admitted the possibility of the new explanation.

11. Eliot Freidson, *Profession of Medicine* (New York: Dodd, Mead, 1974).

1: Getting "Buzzed"

1. U.S. Department of Health, Education, and Welfare, *The Institutional Guide to DHEW Policy on Protection of Human Subjects* (Washington, D.C.: U.S. Government Printing Office, 1971), p. 71.

2. Robert Merton, *Social Theory and Social Structure* (New York: Free Press, 1968), pp. 115–120.

3. When patients dawdle about making a decision they create a power vacuum which physicians readily fill as an exercise in paternalism. Spouses and other family members may also participate in this claim of power. Yet patients may at times find it easier to make a decision when some of the pressure is removed, by the suggestion of outside consultation or support by family or clergy. This is also helpful in situations where the patient, because of fear and stress, may not be competent to handle the decision. It is easy to criticize patients for being irresponsible and failing to make the "right" decision for themselves; yet as long as members of the medical profession continue to make decisions for their patients rather than helping them to make their own decisions, patients will not learn how to take responsibility. It is no accident that one of physicians' chief gripes is the failure of patients to comply with doctor's orders. They fail to see that patients resent their authority and fail to comprehend the need for compliance. If they get worse, they know that physicians will step in and take over as before. Preventive medicine depends on patient responsibility.

4. Paul Ramsey, *The Patient as Person* (New Haven: Yale University Press, 1975).

5. There is some evidence in support of this hypothesis. See Ralph Alfidi, "Informed Consent: A Study of Patient Reaction," *Journal of the American Medical Association,* 216 (1971), 1325–1329; Lawrence Egbert et al., "Reduction of Postoperative Pain by Encouragement and Instruction of Patients: A Study of Doctor-Patient Rapport," *New England Journal of Medicine,* 270 (1964), 825–827; and James Skipper, Jr., and R. C. Leonard, "Children, Stress and Hospitalization: A Field Experiment," *Journal of Health and Social Behavior,* 9 (1968), 275–287.

2: Being Female

1. For a comprehensive look at Mongolism, see Abraham Lilienfeld, *Epidemiology of Mongolism* (Baltimore: Johns Hopkins Press, 1969).

2. For a discussion of sexual behavior among the mentally retarded, along with a comprehensive bibliography, see Judy Hall, "Sexual Behavior," in *Mental Retardation and Developmental Disabilities,* ed. Joseph Wortis (New York: Brunner/Mazel, 1974), vol. 6, pp. 178–212.

3. While my notes do not document how the request for my participation was phrased, my notes and the materials I prepared are organized around legal and not moral issues. As a researcher in the field, I was repeatedly socialized into the behavior of my subjects and may have volunteered "legal materials," knowing that this would elicit a positive response when "moral" issues might not.

4. The eight states are Arkansas, California, Iowa, North Carolina, Pennsylvania, Oregon, Virginia, and Wisconsin.

5. *DHEW Guidelines,* 39 Fed. Reg. 4730 (1974).

6. *Robinson* v. *California,* 370 U.S. 660 (1962).

7. *Relf* v. *Weinberger,* Civil No. 73-1557 (D.D.C. 1974).

8. *Buck* v. *Bell,* 274 U.S. 200 (1927). Justice Holmes concludes that "the principle that sustains compulsory vaccination is broad enough to cover cutting the fallopian tubes."

9. Subsequent landmark decisions limited the scope of *Buck* v. *Bell.* In *Davis* v. *Walton,* 74 Utah 80, 276 Pac. 921 (1929), the Supreme Court of Utah ruled that sterilization is legal only in cases where the "mental insufficiency" is traceable to genetic inheritance and will in all likelihood be transmitted to progeny. *Skinner* v. *Oklahoma,* 316 U.S. 525 (1942), established that "a strict scrutiny" standard of review must be upheld, given that procreation is "a fundamental interest." *Griswold* v. *Connecticut,* 381 U.S. 479 (1965), discussed the nature of family privacy as a basis for invalidating statutory prohibition of birth control devices. This and related cases have contributed to making reproduction an issue of privacy between adults. See also *Eisenstadt* v. *Baird,* 405 U.S. 438 (1972); *Doe* v. *Bolton,* 410 U.S. 179 (1973); and *Roe* v. *Wade,* 410 U.S. 113 (1972).

3: Letting Go

1. An "interesting case," also known as a "fascinoma," is a case of clinical interest because of its complexity of medical management or because of its clinical rarity. These criteria are not appropriate to the medical student in the early phases of his clinical training; for him anything which is a "first"—"my first GI bleed"—is an "interesting case." Students desire the greatest possible variety of medical problems; a run of diabetics ceases to be "interesting."

2. The current debate over the acceptability of "brain death" as the legal criterion of death is exemplified in the following articles: Alexander Capron and Leon Kass, "A Statutory Definition of the Standards for Determining Human Death: An Appraisal and a Proposal," *University of Pennsylvania Law Review,* 121 (1972), 87–118:

Roger Dworkin, "Death in Context," *Indiana Law Journal,* 48 (1973), 623–33; and Robert Morrison, "Death: Process or Event," *Science,* 1873 (1971), 694.

3. *Salvageable* is a horrible objectifying term, like picking over trash to see whether it is worth taking. As Diana Crane demonstrates, determinants of "salvageability" vary with medical services in terms of both clinical and social criteria. See Diana Crane, *The Sanctity of Social Life: Physicians' Treatment of Critically Ill Patients* (New York: Russell Sage Foundation, 1975).

4. William Cannon, "The Right to Die," *Houston Law Review,* 7 (1970), 654–670; Robert Malone, "Is There a Right to a Natural Death?" *New England Law Review,* 9 (Winter 1974), 293–310; and Michael Sullivan, "The Dying Person: His Plight and His Right," *New England Law Review,* 8 (Spring 1973), 197–216. See also Eric Cassell, "Dying in a Technological Society," *Hastings Center Studies,* 2 (May 1974), 31–36.

5. Helpful bibliographies include: Richard Kalish, "Death and Dying: A Briefly Annotated Bibliography," in *The Dying Patient,* ed. Orville Brim, Jr., et al. (New York: Russell Sage Foundation, 1970), pp. 323–380; A. Kutscher, *Bibliography of Books on Death, Bereavement, Loss and Grief: 1955–1968* (New York: Health Sciences Publishing Corp., 1969); U.S. Department of HEW, Public Health Service, National Institute of Health, *Selected Bibliography on Death and Dying,* ed. Joel Vernick (Washington, D.C., 1968). Among more recent publications, see Peter Steinfels and Robert Veatch, *Death Inside Out* (New York: Harper and Row, 1975); Edwin Shneidman, *Death: Current Perspectives* (Palo Alto: Mayfield, 1976); and Robert Veatch, *Death, Dying, and the Biological Revolution* (New Haven: Yale University Press, 1976).

6. For discussion of the distinction between acts of commission and acts of omission, see George Fletcher, "Prolonging Life," *Washington Law Review,* 42 (1967), 999–1016. See also F. D. Moore, "Medical Responsibility for the Prolonging of Life," *Journal of the American Medical Association,* 206 (1968), 384–386; Anthony Shaw, "Dilemmas of 'Informed Consent' in Children," *New England Journal of Medicine,* 289 (October 25, 1973), 885–890; and Jonathan Bennett, "Whatever the Consequences," *Analyses,* 26 (January 1966), 83–102.

7. The problem grows more complicated when the physician believes the patient can get better and will be able to leave the hospital if aggressive therapy is provided, while the patient contends he or she *is dying and wants to die,* or where the patient's family believes that the patient would be better off dead, while the staff still holds hope for recovery. Physicians know that toxicity may contribute to the patient's desire for death; that once the patient's condition improves, he or she will regain the desire to live. A similar argument exists with regard to pain. But should the physician's judgment always take precedence over the patient's? What are the appropriate conditions?

8. Norman Cantor, "A Patient's Decision to Decline Life-Saving Medical Treatment: Bodily Integrity versus the Preservation of Life," *Rutgers Law Review,* 26 (Winter 1972), 228–264.

'9. The record is not totally unambiguous, but certain principles recur. The right to privacy allows one to do with one's body as one sees fit as long as there are no minor dependents requiring the patient's care. Religious freedom may also be admitted as supporting a right to refuse treatment, as well as the rights to bodily integrity and self-determination. Yet the question is never decided in identifiable terms of "a right to die," *per se.* The Quinlan case is a good example. The New Jersey Supreme Court argued: "Nevertheless, we have concluded that Karen's right of privacy may be asserted on her guardian under the peculiar circumstances here present'' (*The New York Times,* April 1, 1976, p. 24).

10. *Union Pacific Railway* v. *Botsford,* 141 U.S. 250, 251 (1891), is generally the earliest cited case. See also *Schloendorff* v. *Society of N.Y. Hosp.,* 211 N.Y. 125, 129–130, 105 N.E. 92, 93 (1914); *Schmerber* v. *California,* 384 U.S. 757 (1966); *In re Yetter,* 62 Pa. D. & C. 2d 619.

11. See note 4. A case to be noted is *Stanley* v. *Georgia,* 394 U.S. 557 (1969).

12. *Zepeda* v. *Zepeda,* 41 Ill. App. 2d 240, 190 N.E. 2d 849 (1963), *cert. denied,* 379 U.S. 945 (1964); and *Williams* v. *New York,* 25 App. Div. 2d 907, 269 N.Y.S. 2d 786 (1966).

13. In *Williams* v. *New York* the argument was used that damages cannot be ascertained because they rest ''upon the very fact of conception.'' For Alexander Capron's criticism of this argument, see ''Informed Decision-Making in Genetic Counseling: A Dissent to the 'Wrongful Life' Debate,'' *Indiana Law Journal,* 48 (1973), 598–604.

14. Lewis Thomas, *The Lives of a Cell: Notes of a Biology Watcher* (New York: Bantam Books, 1975), distinguishes between ''nontechnology,'' ''halfway technology,'' and ''taken-for-granted technology.'' The last consists of the technology of innoculations, antibiotics, chemotherapy—technology based on a genuine understanding of disease mechanisms, which is relatively cheap to produce as well as relatively easy to deliver. The middle term describes the available technology that compensates for existing pathology, for example, transplantations and artificial body parts. It is costly and expensive to deliver. The first consists of the non-measurable—being capable neither of altering the course of disease nor of predicting the outcome. Called ''caring'' or ''bedside manner,'' it is what physicians offer to patients with incurable diseases where there is no compensatory technology.

15. See George Herbert Mead, *Mind, Self, and Society* (Chicago: University of Chicago Press, 1972), p. 171.

16. Jacques Choron, *Death and Western Thought* (New York: Collier Books, 1973).

17. See Paul Ramsey, ''The Indignity of 'Death With Dignity,' '' *Hastings Center Studies,* 2 (May 1974), 47–62, and the commentaries that follow: Robert Morison, ''The Last Poem: The Dignity of the Inevitable and the Necessary,'' 63–66; Leon Kass, ''Averting One's Eyes, or Facing the Music?—On Dignity in Death,'' 67–80.

4: Charting Ethics

1. Talcott Parsons, *The Social System* (New York: Free Press, 1957), pp. 428–479; id., ''The Sick Role and the Role of the Physician Reconsidered,'' *Millbank Memorial Fund Quarterly,* Summer 1975, pp. 257–278.

2. ''[Women] average 25 per cent more visits to the doctor each year than men (100 per cent more if visits of mothers with children are counted); take 50 per cent more prescription drugs than men; and are admitted to hospitals much more frequently than men'' (*Health PAC Bulletin,* March 170, p. 1, quoted in *Our Bodies, Ourselves* [New York: Simon and Schuster, 1976], p. 337).

3. Conversation with Otto Pollak, 1975.

4. The AMA Code (1966) is reprinted, along with the Nuremburg Code (1946–

1949), and the U.S. Public Health Service requirements (December 12, 1966), in Henry Beecher, *Research and the Individual* (Boston: Little, Brown, 1970), pp. 122–127.

5: The Clinical Perspective

1. G. J. Barker-Benfield, "A Historical Perspective on Women's Health Care—Female Circumcision," *Woman and Health,* 1 (January/February 1976), 13–15.

2. Renée Fox and Judith Swazey, *The Courage to Fail* (Chicago: University of Chicago Press, 1974), pp. 122–148.

3. Ibid., pp. 215–217. See also Alan Anderson, Jr., "Dialysis or Death," *New York Times Magazine* (March 7, 1976), pp. 40–48.

4. For a fictional treatment of the problem, including the debate over the "treatment of choice," see Henry Denker, *The Physicians* (New York: Pocket Books, 1975).

5. Rose L. Coser, "Authority and Decision-making in a Hospital: A Comparative Analysis," *American Sociological Review,* 23 (February 1958), pp. 56–63.

6: The Legal Perspective

1. This characterization of the legal process is solely that of the author and a matter not of particular concern to the lawyer. The subsequent discussion is filtered through a sociological perspective and thus does not pretend to legal sophistication. See Peter Berger, *Invitation to Sociology: A Humanistic Perspective* (Garden City, N.Y.: Anchor Books, 1963), pp. 25–53.

2. An example of post-principle law is the judicial concept of "separate but equal" upheld in *Plessy* v. *Ferguson* (163 U.S. 537, 1896) and reversed by *Brown* v. *Board of Education of Topeka* (347 U.S. 483, 1954), in which the Warren Court held that segregation in public education was a denial of equal protection of the laws.

3. The literature on informed consent is abundant. Jon Waltz and Thomas Scheuneman, "Informed Consent to Therapy," *Northwestern University Law Review,* 64 (1969), 628–649, is an excellent introduction to available materials; see footnotes 1 and 3, especially. For informed consent as it pertains to malpractice, see Michael Myers, "Informed Consent in Medical Malpractice," *California Law Review,* 55 (1967), 1396–1418. For a casebook treatment of the issues, see Jay Katz, Alexander Capron, and Eleanor Glass, *Experimentation with Human Beings* (New York: Russell Sage Foundation, 1972), 521–724.

4. *Natanson* v. *Kline,* 186 Kan. 393, 350 P. 2d 1093 (1960). Two other cases sometimes cited as bellwethers of informed consent are *Mitchell* v. *Robinson,* 334 S.W. 2d 11 (Mo. 1960), and *DiFilippo* v. *Preston,* 53 Del. 539, 542, 173 A. 2d 333, 335 (1961).

The citation of specific cases as the historical precedents of *Natanson* v. *Kline* varies from author to author, in part arising from identification of either assault or negligence as the theoretical basis for such a principle. See Katz, *Experimentation with Human Beings,* pp. 524–540; and Myers, "Informed Consent," pp. 1399–41.

See also "Notes: Informed Consent and the Dying Patient," *Yale Law Journal*, 83 (1974), 1633–37.

In *Pratt* v. *Davis*, 118 Ill. App. 161, 166 (1905), affirmed, 224 Ill. 30, 79 N.E. 562 (1906), it was the opinion of the court that "the inviolability of [the] person" forbids a physician or surgeon to perform a major operation requiring total anesthesia without the consent and knowledge of the patient.

See also *Barnett* v. *Bachrach*, 34 A. 2d 626 (D.C. Mun. Ct. App. 1943); and *Bang* v. *Charles T. Miller Hospital*, 251 Minn. 427, 88 N.W. 2d 186 (1958).

5. See Katz, *Experimentation with Human Beings*, p. 554.

6. While most jurisdictions categorize informed consent as either negligence or battery, according to footnote 28 in "Informed Consent and the Dying Patient" (*Yale Law Journal*), Ohio treats it as falling under both theories; see *Belcher* v. *Carter*, 13 Ohio App. 2d 113, 114, 232 N.E. 2d 311, 312 (1967).

For a discussion of the distinction between battery and negligence as arising out of confusion over the theory of recovery, see Stephen Edwards, "Failure to Inform as Medical Malpractice," *Vanderbilt Law Review*, 23 (1970), 754–774. "On the one hand, courts are confronted with the rule: that any treatment administered without the consent of the patient is unauthorized and, therefore, a battery. On the other hand, the ordinary rules of medical malpractice which impose upon the physician a professional standard of care seem applicable to the problem of disclosure" (p. 760). See also Myers, "Informed Consent," notes 16 and 17.

7. Myers, "Informed Consent," p. 1397, cites twenty-two jurisdictions and their standards with regard to these conditions. Edwards distinguishes between express consent of the patient through a written or oral statement of assent (e.g., *Farber* v. *Olkon*, 40 Cal. 2d 503, 254 P. 2d 520 [1953]; *Samuelson* v. *Taylor*, 160 Wash. 369, 295 P. 113 [1931]; consent implied in fact from the patient who demonstrates through his actions that he accepts the recommendations of his physician (e.g., *McGuire* v. *Rix*, 118 Neb. 434, 225 N.W. 120 [1929]); and consent implied in law when the patient because of age or condition is unable to give evidence of his acceptance (e.g., *Luka* v. *Lowrie*, 171 Mich. 122, 136 N.W. 1106 [1912]) ("Failure to Inform," p. 756).

The problems incurred by the patient in obtaining adequate information to fulfill the onditions of "awareness and assent" are discussed within a legal and social perspective by Eleanor Glass, "Notes: Restructuring Informed Consent: Legal Therapy for the Doctor-Patient Relationship," *Yale Law Journal*, 79 (1970), 1533–1576.

8. See, for example, *Roberts* v. *Wood*, 206 F. Supp. 579 (S.D. Ala. 1962); *Valdez* v. *Percy*, 35 Cal. 2d 338, 217 P. 2d 422 (1950); *Natanson* v. *Kline*, 186 Kan. 393, 350 P. 2d 1093 (1960). See Myers, "Informed Consent," pp. 1407–1414; Charles Weyondt, "Comment: Valid Consent to Medical Treatment: Need the Patient Know?" (*Duquesne Law Review*, 450 (1966), 450–462; and Roy Prange, Jr., "Recent Developments in Wisconsin Medical Malpractice Law," *Wisconsin Law Review*, 3 (1974), 893–918.

9. Waltz and Scheuneman, "Informed Consent to Therapy," p. 630. See also ibid., note 25, for the citation of nearly three dozen cases relating to standards of disclosure.

10. For a discussion of the locality rule, see Prange, "Recent Developments" pp. 901–905. For cases discussing the physician's duty as based in the custom and practice of physicians within the community, see, for example, *DiFilippo* v. *Preston*, 53 Del. 539, 173 A. 2d 333 (1961); *Roberts* v. *Young*, 369 Mich. 133, 119 N.W. 2d 627 (1963); *Kaplan* v. *Haines*, 96 N.J. Super. 242, 232 A. 2d 840 (1967); and *Govin* v. *Hunter*, 374 P. 2d—Wyo. (1962).

11. For example, *Ditlow* v. *Kaplan,* 171 So. 2d 225 Fla. App. (1965).

12. For example, *Shetter* v. *Rochelle,* 2 Ariz. App. 358, 409 P. 2d 74 (1965), modified, 2 Ariz. App. 607, 411 P. 2d 45 (1966).

13. Glass, "Restructuring Informed Consent" footnote 67, argues that whether the theory of battery or that of negligence is invoked, the courts require expert testimony to establish liability. The plaintiff carries the burden of establishing a standard of professional behavior and showing some deviation from it. She cites the trend of the courts toward the exclusive use of negligence theory in informed consent litigation.

14. The therapeutic privilege to withhold information from the patient has been discussed in the following cases: *Lester* v. *Aetna Cas. & Sur. Co.,* 240 F. 2d 676, 679 (5th Cir. 1957); *Roberts* v. *Wood,* 206 F. Supp. 579, 583 (S.D. Ala. 1962); *Salgo* v. *Leland Stanford Jr. Univ.,* 154 Cal. App. 2d 560, 578, 317 P. 2d 170, 171 (1957); *Watson* v. *Clutts,* 252 N.C. 153, 159, 136 S.E. 2d 617, 621 (1964).

15. In most cases of fiduciary relationships, the terms of evaluating the fulfillment of professional obligations are not founded on expert testimony by colleagues of the expert. The argument of "community practice" as the determinant of acceptable medical practice is a peculiar one.

16. The courts have generally held that medical testimony must be provided that it is local professional practice to make the disclosure in question before the question of negligence on the part of the physician may be entertained by the jury. So the initial assumption is one of nondisclosure. See Harper and James, Supp. 68, 17.1, n. 15, at 60, cited by Glass, "Restructuring Informed Consent," footnote 96. See also *Hunt* v. *Bradshaw,* 242 N.C. 517, 523, 88 S.E. 2d 762, 766 (1955). Two review articles are Charles Lund, "The Doctor, the Patient and the Truth," *Tennessee Law Review,* 19 (1946), 344–348; and Hubert Smith, "Therapeutic Privilege to Withhold Specific Diagnosis from Patients Sick with Serious or Fatal Illness," *Tennessee Law Review,* 19 (1946), 349–357.

17. The limitation of the same geographic community has been gradually expanded to the "community in which one practices," so that some commentators no longer find it a meaningful concept. See Prange, "Recent Developments," pp. 902–905; *Douglas* v. *Bussabarger,* 73 Wash. 2d 476, 489, 490, 438 P. 2d 829, 837–38 (1968); *Pederson* v. *Dumouchel,* 72 Wash. 2d 73, 77–79, 431, P. 2d 977–78 (1967).

18. The courts have acknowledged this difficulty. See *Christie* v. *Callahan,* 124 F. 2d 825, 828 (D.C. Cir. 1941); *Huffman* v. *Lindquist,* 37 Cal. 2d 465, 484, 234 P. 2d 34, 46 (1951). In *Huffman,* Justice Carter noted, "Anyone familiar with cases of this character knows that the so-called ethical practitioner will not testify on behalf of a plaintiff regardless of the merits of his case." See also "Note: Overcoming the 'Conspiracy of Silence': Statutory and Common Law Innovations," *Minnesota Law Review,* 45 (1961), 1019–1050.

19. Glass, "Restructuring Informed Consent," p. 1558. But therapeutic privilege also undercuts the patient's right to say no, to refuse unwanted treatment, even if from the perspective of the physician it appears to be an irrational and foolish decision. See *Application of the President & Directors of Georgetown College, Inc.,* 118 U.S. App. D.C. 80, 331 F. 2d 1000, *rehearing denied,* 118 U.S. App. D.C. 90, 95–98, 331 P. 2d 1010, 1015–18 (Berger J., dissenting), *cert. denied,* 377 U.S. 978 (1964).

20. William Curran, "Professional Negligence: Some General Comments," *Vanderbilt Law Review,* 12 (1959), 535–547.

21. This is also discussed by Patrick Cassidy, *"Cooper* v. *Roberts:* A 'Reasonable Patient' Test for Informed Consent," *University of Pittsburgh Law Review,* 34 (1973), 500–509. See *Berkey* v. *Anderson,* 1 Cal. App. 3d 790, 82 Cal. Rptr. 67

(1969); *Cooper* v. *Roberts,* 220 Pa. Super. 260, 286 A. 2d 647 (1971); *Canterbury* v. *Spence,* 464 F. 2d 772 (D.C. Cir. 1972); *Wilkinson* v. *Vesey,* 110 R.I. 609, 629, 295 A. 2d 676 (1972); *Hunter* v. *Brown,* 4 Wash. App. 899, 484 P. 2d 1162 (1971).

22. Glass, "Restructuring Informed Consent," footnote 102.

23. See Glass, "Restructuring Informed Consent"; Cassidy, "*Cooper* v. *Roberts*"; Prange, "Recent Developments"; Edwards, "Failure to Inform"; and Myers, "Informed Consent."

24. *Trogun* v. *Fruchtman,* 58 Wis. 2d 569, 207 N.W. 2d 297 (1973); Prange, "Recent Developments."

25. As long as there are no observers who are nonphysicians, the physician has discretionary powers that may be used to resolve legally ambiguous situations. For example, the anesthetized mother cannot witness the physicians' inactivity, which contributes to the death of a deformed newborn, but where "natural childbirth" is the norm, physicians must weigh what the mother (and often the father) will do with respect to their performance. Where observers are other physicians the solidarity of common professional membership protects the physician, even if his actions are professionally, legally, or morally indefensible.

26. Thomas Scheff, "Decision Rules, Types of Error, and Their Consequences in Medical Diagnosis," in *Medical Men and Their Work,* ed. Eliot Freidson and Judith Lorber (Chicago: Aldine, 1975), pp. 309-323.

27. Michel Foucault, *The Birth of the Clinic,* tr. A. M. Sheridan Smith (New York: Pantheon, 1973).

7: The Moral Perspective

1. Alexander Capron, "Informed Decision-Making in Genetic Counseling: A Dissent to the 'Wrongful Life' Debate," *Indiana Law Journal* 48 (Summer 1973), 583-88. See also H. L. A. Hart, "Legal and Moral Obligation," in *Essays in Moral Philosophy,* ed. Abraham Melden (Seattle: University of Washington Press, 1968), pp. 82-107. For another discussion of rights, see Maurice Cranston, *What are Human Rights?* (New York: Taplinger, 1973).

2. See A. V. Campbell, *Moral Dilemmas in Medicine* (Edinburgh: Churchill Livingstone, 1972).

3. "Bibliographe de la sociologie de la vie morale," *Cahiers Internationaux de Sociologie,* 11 (1964), 133-184.

4. I have not attempted to elaborate on the distinctions between "ethics" as a systematic treatment of moral rules and "morals." For those readers who are interested in a discussion of ethics, see Michael Scriven, "The Science of Ethics," pp. 15-43, and Amnon Goldsworth, "Commentary: Utilitarians and the Science of Ethics," pp. 44-48, both in *Science, Ethics and Medicine,* ed. H. Tristam Engelhardt, Jr., and Daniel Callahan (New York: The Hastings Center, 1976).

5. I have found the discussion of moral philosophy in *Moral Problems in Medicine,* ed. Samuel Gorovitz, et al. (Englewood Cliffs, N.J.: Prentice-Hall, 1976) helpful, in particular pp. 12-14.

6. For a series of articles organized around the theme of truth-telling, see Gorovitz, *Moral Problems,* pp. 94-122.

7. For a series of articles organized around the theme of paternalism, see Gorovitz, *Moral Problems,* pp. 182-241.

8. The work of Emile Durkheim is especially representative of these concerns. *The Division of Labor* and *The Elementary Forms of Religious Life* are two of his most famous works.

9. The classic essay on "manifest and latent functions" by Robert Merton, as well as his essays on anomie, demonstrate this orientation. See Robert Merton, *Social Theory and Social Structure,* enl. ed. (New York: Free Press, 1968).

10. See Eike-Henner Kluge, *The Practice of Death* (New Haven: Yale University Press, 1975), pp. 62-63.

11. These extenuating conditions are usually defined as:

1. the act, considered as such as in itself, is not morally bad;
2. the agent's intention in performing the act is directed toward the good effect only;
3. the bad effect is not a necessary and temporally prior means to the good result; and
4. there are grave reasons for considering the act in the first place; reasons of a gravity proportionate to the badness of one of the effects.

Kluge, *Practice of Death,* p. 63.

12. Kluge introduces the doctrine in the context of abortion. See also Philippa Foot, "The Problem of Abortion and the Doctrine of Double Effect," *The Oxford Review,* 1967, pp. 5-15.

13. A developmental model of moral thinking has been the contribution of Lawrence Kohlberg, "Development of Moral Character and Moral Ideology," in *Review of Child Development Research,* ed. Martin Hoffman and Lois Hoffman (New York: Russell Sage Foundation), vol. 1, pp. 383-431.

14. While I have used *universal* in the Parsonian sense (what Parsons identifies as "pattern variables" which describe the orientation of the actor in terms of universalism versus particularism, diffuseness versus specificity, affectivity versus affective neutrality, and ascription versus achievement), Robert Veatch in "Medical Ethics: Professional or Universal?" uses it in the sense of contrasting "universal norms of ethical behavior" with "a special professional ethic" (*Harvard Theological Review,* 65 [1972], 531-559). The interface between the two senses of the term *universal* is intriguing and worth developing.

15. For example, see David Sudnow, *Passing On* (Englewood Cliffs, N.J.: Prentice-Hall, 1967).

16. For additional discussion of the problems of Jehovah's Witnesses as patients, see Laurence Wren, "Status of the Law on Medical and Religious Conflicts in Blood Transfusions," *American Medicine,* 24 (October 1967), 970-973; and George Thomas, Robert Edmark, and Thomas Jones, "Issues Involved with Surgery on Jehovah's Witnesses," *The American Surgeon,* 34 (July 1968), 542-543.

8: The Second-year Student

1. I have used masculine pronouns throughout this section, because the students in the study were all male.

2. T. R. Harrison, Editor-in-Chief, *Harrison's Principles of Internal Medicine,* 7th ed. (New York: McGraw-Hill, 1974), pp. 230-231.

3. Robert Reynolds and Thomas Bice, "Attitudes of Medical Interns toward Pa-

tients and Health Professionals," *Journal of Health and Social Behavior,* 10 (December 1971), 307–311; Allan Schwartzbaum, John McGrath, and Robert Rothman, "The Perception of Prestige Differences Among Medical Subspecialties," *Social Science and Medicine,* 7 (1973), 365–371.

4. Stephen Toulmin, "On the Nature of the Physician's Understanding," *The Journal of Medicine and Philosophy,* 1 (March 1976), 32–50.

5. A. B. Ford et al., "Reaction of Physicians and Medical Students to Chronic Illness," *Journal of Chronic Disease,* 15 (1962), 785–794; William Martin, "Preferences for Types of Patients," in Robert Merton, Patricia Kendall, and George Reader, *The Student Physician,* 2nd ed. (Cambridge, Mass.: Harvard University Press, 1969), pp. 189–206; R. S. Ort et al., "Expectations and Experience in the Reactions of Medical Students to Patients with Chronic Illness," *Journal of Medical Education,* 40 (1965), 840–849; and R. J. Stroller and R. H. Geertsman, "Measurement of Medical Students' Acceptance of Emotionally Ill Patients," *Journal of Medical Education,* 33 (1958), 585–590.

6. Robert Merton, *Social Theory and Social Structure,* enl. ed. (New York: Free Press, 1968), pp. 182–183, 475–490.

7. Agnes Rezler, "Attitude Changes During Medical School: A Review of the Literature," *Journal of Medical Education,* 49 (November 1974), 1371–1375.

8. Robert Lifton, *Thought Reform and the Psychology of Totalism: A Study of "Brainwashing" in China* (New York: Norton, 1961); Joost Meerloo, *The Rape of the Mind: The Psychology of Thought Control, Menticide, and Brainwashing* (New York: Grosset & Dunlap, 1961); and William Sargant, *Battle for the Mind* (New York: Harper and Row, 1971).

9: The Third-year Student

1. There is constant debate about the appropriate use of antibiotics, with the assumption by medical staff members that surgeons prescribe too routinely and with little documentary support for their claims of therapeutic efficacy. See Boyce Rensberger, "Doctors' Scores Low in Test on Use of Antibiotics," *New York Times,* December 18, 1975, p. 30; and Lawrence Altman, "Study Finds that Some Use of Antibiotics May Not Be Justified," *New York Times,* April 8, 1976, p. 24: "A federally funded study in Pennsylvania hospitals has found that 20 percent of the antibiotic drugs prescribed may not be justified by present scientific evidence. . . . This proportion represents the quantity of total antibiotic usage devoted to prophylactic use in surgical patients beyond 48 hours after the operation."

2. Since University Hospital was a "medical man's" hospital, as opposed to a surgeon's, surgeons were generally looked down on as "butchers." (*Intern:* "This place is becoming the training ground for surgeons. . . . There are still a few stupid people who can't do anything else.") Surgeons, however, took pride in their ability to examine a patient, propose surgery, cut the patient open, resolve the problem, sew the patient up, and watch the patient get better without waiting for the positive effects of "slow" methods of treatment. (*Surgical resident:* "If surgeons took care of all your [medical] patients, you'd be out of work.")

3. When the student becomes responsible for working up admissions he becomes concerned with questions like how many patients, how closely spaced, how sick, what

variety of admitting complaint, who admitted the patient, and how many admissions have other services received. If you are on at night you want someone who is not too sick, with an uncomplicated history, with a knowledgeable admitting physician who has previously screened the patient, who is articulate, and who is not accompanied by a hysterical family.

4. "Munchausen" are the bane of the cardiologist's existence. They turn up in city emergency rooms with well-rehearsed histories and symptoms. Once admitted, if they believe they are under suspicion as frauds, they will sign out "against medical advice." See Patricia Ireland et al., "Munchausen's Syndrome," *American Journal of Medicine,* 43 (October 1967), 579–592; Bertrand Cramer et al., "Munchausen Syndrome," *Archives of General Psychiatry,* 24 (June 1971), 573–578; and Milo Tyndel and John Rutherdale, "The Hospital Addiction (Munchausen) Syndrome and Alcoholism," *The International Journal of the Addictions,* 8 (1973), 121–126.

5. The house staff tends to note when elderly men are exceptionally active for their years: climb mountains, do physical labor, and so on, and they may include this in their opening statement. It tends to enhance the aggressiveness of medical efforts on their behalf. Women, however, rarely demonstrate such claims of viability; thus, they are left with the power of charming personality. Patients who are well liked tend to get more aggressive attention than those who are actively disliked.

6. See Harold Lief and Renée Fox, "Training for Detached Concern in Medical Students," in Lief, *Psychological Basis of Medical Practice* (New York: Harper and Row, 1963), pp. 12–35.

10: The Fourth-year Student

1. Thomas Scheff, "Decision Rules, Types of Error, and Their Consequences in Medical Diagnoses," in *Medical Men and Their Work,* ed. Eliot Freidson and Judith Lorber (Chicago: Aldine, 1975), pp. 309–323.

11: Delegation and Autonomy

1. For a parallel, see Curtis Berger, "The Heart of the Law Is the Heart of the Lawyer," *New York Times,* July 6, 1976, p. 25: "Above all, I think that we as teachers must let our students know that we value their humane as well as intellectual qualities—and our own as well as theirs. For unless lawyers value the compassionate in themselves, I think they will be incapable of caring about the human needs of others."

2. For an interesting parallel with this argument regarding the role of sociologists and value judgments, see Alvin Gouldner, "Anti-Minotaur: The Myth of Value-Free Sociology," in *Sociology: Introductory Readings in Mass, Class, and Bureaucracy,* ed. Joseph Beusman and Bernard Rosenberg (New York: Praeger, 1975), p. 50.

3. The problem of autonomy is given full treatment in Eliot Friedson, *Profession of Medicine* (New York: Dodd, Mead, 1974).

4. "Highly Trained Called Targets of Malpractice Claims," *New York Times,* May

10, 1976, p. 23. The study of malpractice claims was prepared by the Association of Insurance Commissioners.

5. David S. Rubsamin, "Medical Malpractice," *Scientific American,* 235 (August 1976), 18-23.

12: Conclusion

1. "Doctors Are Slow to Accept Non-Doctor Assistants," *New York Times,* May 11, 1976, p. 10.

Bibliography

Alfidi, Ralph. "Informed Consent: A Study of Patient Reaction." *Journal of the American Medical Association,* 216 (May 24, 1971), 1325-1329.

Altman, Lawrence. "Study Finds that Some Use of Antibiotics May Not Be Justified." *New York Times,* April 8, 1976, p. 24.

Anderson, Alan, Jr., "Dialysis or Death." *New York Times Magazine,* March 7, 1976, pp. 40-48.

Barber, Bernard. "The Ethics of Experimentation with Human Subjects." *Scientific American,* 234 (February 1976), 25-31.

Barber, Bernard, and Fox, Renée. "The Case of the Floppy-Eared Rabbits: An Instance of Serendipity Gained and Serendipity Lost." *The American Journal of Sociology,* 18 (September 1958), 128-136.

Barker-Benfield, G. J. "A Historical Perspective on Women's Health Care—Female Circumcision." *Women and Health,* 1 (January/February 1976), 13-15.

Becker, Howard; Geer, Blanche; Hughes, Everett; and Strauss, Anselm. *Boys in White: Student Culture in Medical School.* Chicago: University of Chicago Press, 1961.

Becker, Howard. "Problems in Inference and Proof in Participant Observation." *American Sociological Review,* 23 (December 1958), 652-660.

———. *Sociological Work.* Chicago: Aldine, 1970.

Beecher, Henry. *Research and the Individual.* Boston: Little, Brown, 1970.

Berger, Curtis. "The Heart of the Law Is the Heart of the Lawyer." *New York Times,* July 6, 1976, p. 25.

"Bibliographie de la sociologie de la vie morale." *Cahiers Internationaux de sociologie,* 11 (1964), 133-184.

Bloom, Samuel. "The Process of Becoming a Physician." *The Annals of the American Academy of Political and Social Science* 75 (March 1969), 78-82.

Bowen, Elenore Smith [Laura Bohannon]. *Return to Laughter.* Garden City, N.Y.: Anchor Books, 1964.

Brill, Howard. "Death with Dignity: A Recommendation for Statutory Change." *University of Florida Law Review* 22 (Winter 1970), 368–383.

Brim, Orville, Jr., and Wheeler, Stanton. *Socialization after Childhood: Two Essays.* New York: John Wiley and Sons, 1966.

Brooks, Harvey. "Technology and Values: New Ethical Issues Raised by Technological Progress." *Zygon,* 8 (March 1973), 17–35.

Campbell, A. V. *Moral Dilemmas in Medicine.* Edinburgh: Churchill Livingstone, 1972.

Cannon, William. "The Right to Die." *Houston Law Review,* 7 (May 1970), 654–670.

Cant, Gilbert. "Valiumania." *New York Times Magazine,* February 1, 1976, 34–44.

Cantor, Norman. "A Patient's Decision to Decline Life-Saving Medical Treatment: Bodily Integrity versus the Preservation of Life." *Rutgers Law Review* 26 (Winter 1972), 228–264.

Capron, Alexander. "Informed Decision-Making in Genetic Counseling: A Dissent to the 'Wrongful Life' Debate." *Indiana Law Journal,* 48 (Summer 1973), 581–604.

Carmody, James. *Ethical Issues in Health Services: A Report and Annotated Bibliography.* Washington, D.C.: U.S. Department of Health, Education, and Welfare, 1974.

Carr-Saunders, A. M., and Wilson, P. A. *The Professions.* Oxford: Clarendon Press, 1933.

Cassell, Eric. "Dying in a Technological Society." *Hastings Center Studies,* 2 (May 1974), 31–36.

————. *The Healer's Art.* Philadelphia: J. B. Lippincott, 1976.

Cassidy, Patrick Sean. "Cooper v. Roberts: A 'Reasonable Patient' Test for Informed Consent." *University of Pittsburgh Law Review* 34 (Spring 1973), 500–509.

Choron, Jacques. *Death and Western Thought.* New York: Collier Books, 1973.

Clausen, John, ed. *Socialization and Society.* Boston: Little Brown, 1968.

Clouser, K. Danner. "Medical Ethics: Some Uses, Abuses and Limitations." *The New England Journal of Medicine,* 293 (August 21, 1975), 384–387.

Coe, Rodney. *Sociology of Medicine.* New York: McGraw-Hill, 1970.

Cogan, Morris. "The Problem of Defining a Profession." *The Annals of the American Academy of Political and Social Science* 61 (January 1955), 105–111.

————. "Toward a Definition of Profession." *Harvard Educational Review,* 32 (Winter 1953), 33–49.

Cottrell, Leonard, and Sheldon, Eleanor. "Problems of Collaboration between Social Scientists and the Practicing Professions." *The Annals of the American Academy of Political and Social Science,* 66 (March 1963), 126–137.

Crane, Diana. *The Sanctity of Social Life: Physicians' Treatment of Critically Ill Patients.* New York: Russell Sage, 1975.

Cranston, Maurice. *What Are Human Rights?* New York: Taplinger, 1973.

Curran, William. "Professional Negligence: Some General Comments." *Vanderbilt Law Review,* 12 (June 1959), 535–547.

Davies, James. "Toward a Theory of Revolution." *American Sociological Review,* 27, (1962), 5–19.

"Doctors Are Slow to Accept Non-Doctor Assistants." *New York Times* May 11, 1976, p. 10.

Dreitzel, Peter, ed. *Recent Sociology.* No. 2. New York: Macmillan, 1970.

Edwards, Stephen. "Failure to Inform as Medical Malpractice." *Vanderbilt Law Review,* 23 (May 1970), 754–774.

Egbert, Lawrence, et al. "Reduction of Postoperative Pain by Encouragement and Instruction of Patients: A Study of Doctor-Patient Rapport." *New England Journal of Medicine,* 270 (April 16, 1964), 825–827.

Elliott, Philip. *Sociology of the Professions.* London: Macmillan, 1972.

Eron, Leonard. "Effect of Medical Education on Medical Students' Attitudes." *Journal of Medical Education,* 30 (October 1955), 559–566.

Etzioni, Amitai, ed. *The Semi-Professions and Their Origin: Teachers, Nurses, Social Workers.* New York: The Free Press, 1969.

Fletcher, Colin. *Beneath the Surface: An Account of Three Styles of Sociological Research.* London: Routledge and Kegan Paul, 1974.

Fletcher, George. "Legal Aspects of the Decision Not to Prolong Life." *Journal of the American Medical Association* 203 (January 1, 1968), 65–68.

———. "Prolonging Life." *Washington Law Review,* 42 (1967), 999–1016.

Fletcher, John. "Who Should Teach Medical Ethics?" *Hastings Center Report,* 1 (December 1973), 4–6.

Ford, A. B., et al. "Reaction of Physicians and Medical Students to Chronic Illness." *Journal of Chronic Disease, 15 (August 1962), 785–794.*

Foucault, Michael. *The Birth of the Clinic: An Archaeology of Medical Perception.* New York: Pantheon, 1973.

Fox, Renée. *Experiment Perilous: Physicians and Patients Facing the Unknown.* Philadelphia: University of Pennsylvania Press, 1974.

———. "Is There a 'New' Medical Student?" *The Key Reporter,* 30 (Summer 1975), 2–4.

Fox, Renée, and Swazey, Judith. *The Courage to Fail.* Chicago: University of Chicago Press, 1974.

Freeman, Howard, et al., Eds. *Handbook of Medical Sociology.* Englewood Cliffs, N.J.: Prentice-Hall, 1965.

Freidson, Eliot. *Profession of Medicine: A Study of Applied Knowledge.* New York: Dodd, Mead, 1974.

Freidson, Eliot, and Lorber, Judith, eds. *Medical Men and Their Work.* Chicago: Aldine, 1975, pp. 309–323.

Fried, Charles. *Medical Experimentation*. New York: Elsevier, 1974.

Garfinkel, Harold. *Studies in Ethnomethodology*. Englewood Cliffs, N.J.: Prentice-Hall, 1967.

Geertz, Clifford. "Thinking as a Moral Act: Ethical Dimensions of Anthropological Fieldwork in the New States." *Antioch Review,* 28 (1968), 139–158.

Gerth, H. H., and Mills, C. Wright, eds. *From Max Weber*. New York: Oxford University Press, 1970.

Glass, Eleanor. "Notes: Restructuring Informed Consent: Legal Therapy for the Doctor-Patient Relationship." *Yale Law Journal,* 79 (July 1970), 1533–1576.

Goffman, Erving. *Presentation of Self in Everyday Life*. Garden City, N.Y.: Anchor Books, 1959.

Goodman, W. "Doctor's Image Is Sickly." *New York Times Magazine,* October 16, 1966, pp. 38–39.

Gorovitz, Samuel et al. *Moral Problems in Medicine*. Englewood Cliffs, N.J.: Prentice-Hall, 1976.

Gorovitz, Samuel, and MacIntyre, Alasdair. "Toward a Theory of Medical Fallibility." *The Journal of Medicine and Philosophy,* 1 (March 1976), 51–71.

Goss, Mary. "Collaboration between Sociologist and Physician." *Social Problems,* 11 (July 1956), 82–89.

Gould, D. "Power and Sickness." *The New Statesman,* 21 (July 7, 1967), 13.

Gouldner, Alvin. "Anti-Minotaur: The Myth of Value-Free Sociology." In Bensman, Joseph, and Rosenberg, Bernard. *Sociology: Introductory Readings in Mass, Class, and Bureaucracy*. New York: Praeger, 1975, pp. 45–58.

Gouldner, Alvin. "Cosmopolitans and Locals: Toward an Analysis of Latent Social Roles." *Administrative Science Quarterly,* 45 (December 1957), 281–306.

Habenstein, Robert. "Critique of 'Profession' as a Sociological Category." *Sociology Quarterly,* 51 (Autumn 1963), 298–300.

Hammond, Philip, ed. *Sociologists at Work*. New York: Basic Books, 1964.

Harrison, T. R., et al., eds. *Harrison's Principles of Internal Medicine*. 7th ed. New York: McGraw-Hill, 1974.

"Highly Trained Called Targets of Malpractice Claims." *New York Times,* May 10, 1976, p. 23.

Hughes, Everett. "The Making of a Physician." *Human Organization,* 15 (Winter 1955), 21–24.

Ingelfinger, Franz. "The Unethical in Medical Ethics." *Annals of Internal Medicine,* 83 (August 1975), 264–269.

Ireland, Patricia, et al. "Munchausen's Syndrome." *American Journal of Medicine,* 261 (October 1967), 579–592.

Jackson, J. A., ed. *Professions and Professionalization*. Cambridge: Cambridge University Press, 1970.

Jaco, E. Garly, ed. *Patients, Physicians and Illness*. New York: Free Press, 1958.

Johnson, John, Jr., "An Evaluation of Changes in the Medical Standard of Care." *Vanderbilt Law Review,* 23 (May 1970), 129–153.

Jones, W. H. S. *The Doctor's Oath: An Essay in the History of Medicine*. Cambridge: The University Press, 1924.

Katz, Jay; Capron, Alexander; and Glass, Eleanor. *Experimentation with Human Beings*. New York: Russell Sage Foundation, 1972.

Kübler-Ross, Elizabeth. *On Death and Dying*. New York: MacMillan, 1969.

Larned, Deborah. "Do You Take Valium?" *Ms. Magazine,* 4 (November 1975), 26–28.

Lief, Harold and Fox, Renée, "The Medical Student's Training for Detached Concern." In Lief, H. I., et al. *The Psychological Basis of Medical Practice*. New York: Harper and Row, 1963, pp. 12–35.

Lifton, Robert. *Thought Reform and the Psychology of Totalism: A Study of "Brainwashing" in China*. New York: Norton, 1961.

Lilienfield, Abraham. *Epidemiology of Mongolism*. Baltimore: Johns Hopkins Press, 1969.

Lund, Charles. "The Doctor, the Patient, and the Truth." *Tennessee Law Review,* 19 (1946), 344–48.

McCall, George, and Simmons, J. L. *Issues in Participant Observation*. Reading, Mass.: Addison-Wesley, 1969.

McKinlay, J. B. "Who Is Really Ignorant—Physician or Patient?" *Journal of Health and Social Behavior,* 16 (March 1975), 3–11.

Malone, Robert. "Is There a Right to a Natural Death?" *New England Law Review,* 9 (Winter 1974), 293–310.

Markowitz, G. E., and Rosner, D. K. "Doctors in Crisis: A Study of the Use of Educational Reform to Establish Modern Professional Elitism in Medicine." *American Quarterly,* 61 (March 1973), 83–107.

Mead, George Herbert. *Mind, Self, and Society*. Chicago: University of Chicago Press, 1972.

Mechanic, David. *Medical Sociology: A Selective View*. New York: Free Press, 1968.

Meerloo, Joost. *The Rape of the Mind: The Psychology of Thought Control, Menticide, and Brainwashing*. New York: Grosset and Dunlap, 1961.

Melden, Abraham, ed. *Essays in Moral Philosophy*. Seattle: University of Washington Press, 1968.

Merton, Robert. *Social Theory and Social Structure*. Enl. ed. New York: Free Press, 1968.

Merton, Robert; Kendall, Patricia; and Reader, George, eds. *The Student Physician*. 2nd ed. Cambridge, Mass.: Harvard University Press, 1969.

Moore, F. D. "Medical Responsibility for the Prolonging of Life." *Journal of the American Medical Association,* 206 (1968), 384–386.

Moore, W. E. *The Professions: Roles and Rules*. New York: Russell Sage Foundation, 1970.

Mumford, Emily, and Skipper, J. K. *Sociology in Hospital Care*. New York: Harper and Row, 1967.

Myerhoff, Barbara, and Larson, William. "The Doctor As Culture Hero: The Routinization of Charisma." *Human Organization*, 24 (Fall 1965), 188-191.

Myers, Michael. "Informed Consent in Medical Malpractice." *California Law Review*, 55 (November 1967), 1396-1418.

National Library of Medicine. "Attitudes Toward Death." *Literature Search No. 71-4* (January 1968—March 1971). Washington, D.C.: U.S. Department of Health, Education, and Welfare, 1971.

"Note: Overcoming the 'Conspiracy of Silence': Statutory and Common Law Innovations." *Minnesota Law Review*, 45 (1961), 1019-1050.

"Notes: Informed Consent and the Dying Patient." *Yale Law Journal*, 83 (July 1974), 1633-1637.

Olesen, Virginia, and Whittaker, Elvi. "Role-Making in Participant Observation: Processes in the Researcher-Actor Relationship." *Human Organization*, 24 (Winter 1967), 273-281.

Ort, R. S., et al. "Expectations and Experience in the Reactions of Medical Students to Patients with Chronic Illness." *Journal of Medical Education*, 40 (September 1965), 840-849.

Parsons, Talcott. "The Sick Role and the Role of the Physician Reconsidered." *Millbank Memorial Fund Quarterly*, Summer 1975, 257-278.

————. *The Social System*. New York: Free Press, 1951.

Pellegrino, Edmund. "Educating the Humanist Physician." *Journal of the American Medical Association*, 227 (March 18, 1974), 1288-1294.

Percival, Thomas. *Percival's Medical Ethics*. Edited by Chauncey Leake. Baltimore: Williams and Wilkins, 1927.

"Physician Warns about Incompetent Doctors." *U.S. News and World Report*, 60 (January 3, 1966), 10.

"Physician, What Ails Thee?" *Newsweek*, 84 (October 18, 1971), 84.

Prange, Roy, Jr., "Recent Developments in Wisconsin Medical Malpractice Law." *Wisconsin Law Review*, 3 (1974), 893-918.

Rainwater, Lee, and Pittman, David. "Ethical Problems in Studying a Politically Sensitive and Deviant Community." *Social Problems*, 14 (Spring 1967), 357-366.

Ramsey, Paul. "The Indignity of 'Death with Dignity.' " *Hastings Center Studies*, 2 (May 1974), 47-62.

————. *The Patient as Person*. New Haven: Yale University Press, 1975.

Rensberger, Boyce. "Doctors' Scores Low in Test on Use of Antibiotics." *New York Times*, December 18, 1975, p. 30.

Reynolds, Paul. "Value Dilemmas in the Professional Conduct of Social Science." *International Social Journal*, 27 (1975), 563–627.

Reynolds, Robert, and Brice, Thomas. "Attitudes of Medical Interns Toward Patients and Health Professionals." *Journal of Health and Social Behavior*, 10 (December 1971), 307–311.

Rezler, Agnes. "Attitude Changes During Medical School: A Review of the Literature." *Journal of Medical Education*, 49 (November 1974), 1371–1375.

Rubsamin, David S. "Medical Malpractice," *Scientific American*, 235 (August 1976), 18–23.

Russell Sage Foundation. *Annual Report*, Vols. 59, 64. New York: Russell Sage Foundation, 1958, 1963.

"Rx from the Patient: Physician, Heal Thyself." *Time*, 88 (May 13, 1966), 46–47.

Sargant, William. *Battle for the Mind*. New York: Harper and Row, 1971.

Schatzman, Leonard, and Strauss, Anselm. *Field Research: Strategies for a Natural Sociology*. Englewood Cliffs, N.J.: Prentice-Hall, 1973.

Schlick, Moritz. *Problems of Ethics*. Translated by David Rynin, New York: Dover Publications, 1962.

Schwartzbaum, Allan; McGrath, John; and Rothman, Robert. "The Perception of Prestige Differences Among Medical Specialties." *Social Science and Medicine*, 7 (1973), 365–371.

Scott, W. Richard, and Volkart, Edmund, eds. *Medical Care: Readings in the Sociology of Medical Institutions*. New York: John Wiley and Sons, 1966.

Shaw, Anthony. "Dilemmas of 'Informed Consent' in Children." *New England Journal of Medicine*, 289 (October 25, 1973), 885–890.

Silverman, M. "Can We Get Rid of Bad Doctors?" *Saturday Evening Post*, 243 (Summer 1971), 19.

Skipper, James, Jr., and Leonard, R. C. "Children, Stress and Hospitalization: A Field Experiment." *Journal of Health and Social Behavior*, 9 (1968), 275–287.

Smith, Hubert. "Therapeutic Privilege to Withhold Specific Diagnosis from Patients Sick with Serious or Fatal Illness." *Tennessee Law Review*, 19 (1946), 349–357.

Straus, Robert. "A Role for Behavioral Science in a University Medical Center." *The Annals of the American Academy of Political and Social Science*, 67 (March 1963), 99–108.

Stroller, R. J., and Geertsman, R. H. "Measurement of Medical Students' Acceptance of Emotionally Ill Patients." *Journal of Medical Education*, 33 (August 1958), 585–590.

Sudnow, David. *Passing On*. Englewood Cliffs, N.J.: Prentice-Hall, 1967.

Sullivan, Michael. "The Dying Person: His Plight and His Right." *New England Law Review*, 8 (Spring 1973), 197–216.

Susser, M. W., and Watson, W. *Sociology in Medicine*. London: Oxford University Press, 1962.

Thomas, Lewis. *The Lives of a Cell: Notes of a Biology Watcher*. New York: Bantam Books, 1975.

Toulmin, Stephen. *Human Understanding*. Princeton: Princeton University Press, 1972.

————. "On the Nature of the Physician's Understanding." *The Journal of Medicine and Philosophy*, 1 (March 1976), 32–50.

Turner, Roy, ed. *Ethnomethodology*. Baltimore: Penguin Books, 1974, pp. 15–18.

U.S. Department of Health, Education, and Welfare. *The Institutional Guide to DHEW Policy on Protection of Human Subjects*. Washington, D.C.: U.S. Government Printing Office, 1971.

Veatch, Robert, and Clouser, Danner. "New Mix in the Medical Curriculum." *Prism*, 1 (November 1973), 62–66.

Veatch, Robert, and Gaylin, Willard. "Teaching Medical Ethics: An Experimental Program." *Journal of Medical Education*, 47 (October 1972), 779–785.

Veith, Ilza. "Medical Ethics Throughout the Ages." *Archives of Internal Medicine*, 100 (1957), 504–512.

Vidich, Arthur, and Bensman, Joseph. *Small Town in Mass Society*. Rev. ed. Princeton: Princeton University Press, 1970, pp. 397–476.

Vidich, Arthur; Bensmann, Joseph; and Stein, Maurice, eds. *Reflections on Community Studies*. New York: John Wiley, 1964, pp. 267–284.

Vollmer, Howard. *Professionalization*. Englewood Cliffs, N.J.: Prentice-Hall, 1966.

Walters, LeRoy. *Bibliography of Bio-ethics*. Vol. 1. Detroit: Gale Research, 1975.

Waltz, Jon, and Scheuneman, Thomas. "Informed Consent to Therapy." *Northwestern University Law Review*, 64 (November–December 1969), 628–649.

Wax, Rosalie. "Reciprocity As a Field Technique." *Human Organization*, 11 (Fall 1952), 34–37.

Index